Specialty Competencies
in Geropsychology

Series in Specialty Competencies in Professional Psychology

TITLES IN THE SERIES

Specialty Competencies in School Psychology, Rosemary Flanagan and Jeffrey A. Miller

Specialty Competencies in Organizational and Business Consulting Psychology, Jay Thomas

Specialty Competencies in Geropsychology, Victor Molinari (Ed.)

EDITED BY
VICTOR MOLINARI

Specialty Competencies
in Geropsychology

OXFORD
UNIVERSITY PRESS

2011

OXFORD
UNIVERSITY PRESS

Oxford University Press, Inc., publishes works that further
Oxford University's objective of excellence
in research, scholarship, and education.

Oxford New York

Auckland   Cape Town   Dar es Salaam   Hong Kong   Karachi
Kuala Lumpur   Madrid   Melbourne   Mexico City   Nairobi
New Delhi   Shanghai   Taipei   Toronto

With offices in
Argentina   Austria   Brazil   Chile   Czech Republic   France   Greece
Guatemala   Hungary   Italy   Japan Poland   Portugal   Singapore
South Korea   Switzerland   Thailand   Turkey   Ukraine   Vietnam

Copyright © 2011 by Oxford University Press, Inc.

Published by Oxford University Press, Inc.
198 Madison Avenue, New York, New York 10016
www.oup.com

Oxford is a registered trademark of Oxford University Press

CIP on file

ISBN 9780195385670 Paper

9 8 7 6 5 4 3 2 1

Printed in the United States of America
on acid-free paper

ABOUT THE SERIES IN SPECIALTY COMPETENCIES IN PROFESSIONAL PSYCHOLOGY

This series is intended to describe state-of-the-art functional and foundational competencies in professional psychology across extant and emerging specialty areas. Each book in this series provides a guide to best practices across both core and specialty competencies as defined by a given professional psychology specialty.

The impetus for this series was created by various growing movements in professional psychology during the past 15 years. First, as an applied discipline, psychology is increasingly recognizing the unique and distinct nature among a variety of orientations, modalities, and approaches with regard to professional practice. These specialty areas represent distinct ways of practicing one's profession across various domains of activities that are based on distinct bodies of literature and often addressing differing populations or problems. For example, the American Psychological Association (APA) in 1995 established the Commission on the Recognition of Specialties and Proficiencies in Professional Psychology (CRSPPP) in order to define criteria by which a given specialty could be recognized. The Council of Credentialing Organizations in Professional Psychology (CCOPP), an inter-organizational entity, was formed in reaction to the need to establish criteria and principles regarding the types of training programs related to the education, training, and professional development of individuals seeking such specialization. In addition, the Council on Specialties in Professional Psychology (CoS) was formed in 1997, independent of the APA, to foster communication among the established specialties, in order to offer a unified position to the pubic regarding specialty education and training, credentialing, and practice standards across specialty areas.

Simultaneously, efforts to actually define professional competence regarding psychological practice have also been growing significantly. For example, the APA-sponsored Task Force on Assessment of Competence in Professional Psychology put forth a series of guiding principles for the assessment of competence within professional psychology, based, in part, on a review of competency assessment models developed both within (e.g., Assessment of Competence Workgroup from Competencies Conference— Roberts et al., 2005) and outside (e.g., Accreditation Council for Graduate Medical Education and American Board of Medical Specialties, 2000) the profession of psychology (Kaslow et al., 2007).

Moreover, additional professional organizations in psychology have provided valuable input into this discussion, including various associations primarily interested in the credentialing of professional psychologists, such as the American Board of Professional Psychology (ABPP), the Association of State and Provincial Psychology Boards (ASPBB), and the National Register of Health Service Providers in Psychology. This wide-spread interest and importance of the issue of competency in professional psychology can be especially appreciated given the attention and collaboration afforded to this effort by international groups, including the Canadian Psychological Association and the International Congress on Licensure, Certification, and Credentialing in Professional Psychology.

Each volume in the series is devoted to a specific specialty and provides a definition, description, and development timeline of that specialty, including its essential and characteristic pattern of activities, as well as its distinctive and unique features. Each set of authors, long-term experts and veterans of a given specialty, were asked to describe that specialty along the lines of both functional and foundational competencies. *Functional competencies* are those common practice activities provided at the specialty level of practice that include, for example, the application of its science base, assessment, intervention, consultation, and where relevant, supervision, management, and teaching. *Foundational competencies* represent core knowledge areas which are integrated and cut across all functional competencies to varying degrees, and dependent upon the specialty, in various ways. These include ethical and legal issues, individual and cultural diversity considerations, interpersonal interactions, and professional identification.

Whereas we realize that each specialty is likely to undergo changes in the future, we wanted to establish a baseline of basic knowledge and principles that comprise a specialty highlighting both its commonalities with other areas of professional psychology, as well as its distinctiveness. We look forward to seeing the dynamics of such changes, as well as the emergence of new specialties in the future.

The current volume describes the foundational and functional competencies underlying "geropsychology," the area in professional psychology that focuses on the psychological and behavioral aspects of aging. Officially,

CRSPPP had designated "clinical geropsychology" as a proficiency in professional psychology in 1998, rather than as a "specialty." However, we decided to include this subfield within our series due to the burgeoning demand for competent psychological services likely to occur in the near future as a function of the aging of the population within the United States. Indeed, it may be considered a specialty within the next few years. Note that a slight deviation from other volumes in this series is its structure. Based in large part on the Pikes Peak model for training in professional geropsychology, this book includes multiple chapter authors under the expert editorship of Victor Molinari. As described in chapter 1, "the ultimate goal of geropsychology is to apply scientific findings about psychological aging to improve the lives of older adults." We believe that psychologists interested in working with older adults will find this volume both educational and aspirational.

Arthur M. Nezu
Christine Maguth Nezu

References Cited

Kaslow, N. J., Rubin, N. J., Bebeau, M. J., Leigh, I. W., Lichtenberg, J. W., Nelson, P. D., Portnoy, S. M., & Smith, I. L. (2007). Guiding principles and recommendations for the assessment of competence. *Professional Psychology: Research and Practice, 38*, 441–451.

Roberts, M. C., Borden, K. A., Christiansen, M. D., & Lopez, S. J. (2005). Fostering a culture shift: Assessment of competence in the education and careers of professional psychologists. *Professional Psychology: Research and Practice, 36*, 355–361.

ACKNOWLEDGMENTS

I take this opportunity to acknowledge all the attendees at the June 2006 National Conference on Training in Professional Geropsychology (Pikes Peak conference) who devoted their time and energy to make it so successful and who developed the training model that is the cornerstone for the chapters in this volume.

Victor Molinari

CONTENTS

CONTRIBUTORS

Barry Edelstein, PhD
West Virginia University
Morgantown, WV

Erin Emery, PhD
Rush University Medical Center
Chicago, IL

Gregory A. Hinrichsen, PhD
Albert Einstein College of
    Medicine
Bronx, NY

Michele J. Karel, PhD
Brockton VA Medical Center
Brockton, MA

Lesley Koven, PhD
University of Manitoba
Winnipeg, Manitoba
CANADA

Victor Molinari, PhD, ABPP
University of South Florida
Tampa, FL

Andrew Presnell, MA
University of Alabama
Tuscaloosa, AL

Sara Honn Qualls, PhD
University of Colorado at
    Colorado Springs
Colorado Springs, CO

Forrest Scogin, PhD
University of Alabama
Tuscaloosa, AL

Yvette N. Tazeau, PhD
YNT Consulting
San Jose, CA

Tammi Vacha-Haase, PhD
Colorado State University
Fort Collins, CO

Susan Krauss Whitbourne, PhD
University of Massachusetts
    Amherst
Amherst, MA

Lauren A. Zeranski, BA
University of Massachusetts
    Amherst
Amherst, MA

INTRODUCTION

In the fall of 2008, I was approached by Drs. Arthur and Christine Nezu about writing a volume on competencies in geropsychology for their well regarded "Series on Specialty Competencies in Professional Psychology, published by Oxford University Press". Although I was honored to be asked to be the author of this book, I was very much aware that the knowledge base and clinical applications in clinical geropsychology have so much progressed over the years that I would not be able to do justice to all the topics that needed to be covered. Happily, the Pikes Peak conference had convened in the summer of 2006 and the proceedings were still fresh in the minds of its participants. Responsive to my predicament, a number of these experts readily agreed to write chapters in an edited book format.

Professional Competencies in Geropsychology is the fruit of the toils of their labor (and indeed of all the prior training guidelines and conferences that paved the way for the Pikes Peak conference), and I expect that the readers will be as pleased as I am with the final result. In a way, this book is a more detailed follow-up on a series of recent papers that have been published (Hinrichsen, Zeiss, Karel & Molinari, 2010; Karel, Knight, Duffy, Hinrichsen, & Zeiss, 2010; Knight, Karel, Hinrichsen, Qualls, & Duffy, 2009), regarding the products of the Pikes Peak conference. Its purpose is to describe the knowledge, skill, and attitude competencies that individuals should possess to consider themselves clinical geropsychologists. This book is divided into three parts based on these three main competencies. As the editor, I recognize that these competencies are intrinsically interrelated, and acknowledge that this partitioning was performed for didactic ends.

In the first chapter, I attempt to highlight the past accomplishments of professional geropsychology to serve as a guidepost for emerging initiatives regarding the further refinement of knowledge, skill, and attitude competencies. Just as the life review literature reminds us that gaining perspective on the past will allow us to understand where we have been, to recognize what else needs to be accomplished, and thereby to inform future endeavors, my hope is that this chapter will allow us to pause and take stock of our professional identity in this critical period of our development.

In the next two chapters of Part I, knowledge competencies are detailed. Drs. Qualls and Whitbourne set the stage for an understanding of the foundational competencies of geropsychology and their historical roots in the painstaking basic research of life span development. Dr. Qualls is well acquainted with the historical tradition of geropsychology and has coordinated an annual conference in geropsychology for a number of years. Dr. Whitbourne is nationally known for her well respected textbooks that are fine exemplars of applying developmental understanding in clinical work with older adults.

In Part II, skill competencies are addressed. Drs. Edelstein, Hinrichsen, Scogin, and Emery are the primary authors for these chapters that outline the use of basic understanding of gerontological processes for the bio-psycho-social assessment, treatment, and consultation with older adults. As dynamic clinicians, applied researchers, and sage mentor/teachers, these authors are able to merge theory and practice while remaining 'experience near', eschewing sterile theorizing in favor of tackling the hard clinical realities of practitioners in the geriatric trenches.

In Part III, attitude competencies are discussed. Drs. Tazeau, Karel, and Vacha-Haase tackle the thorny professional issues of multicultural competency, decision-making when faced with ethical quandaries, and the training of future professionals for careers in geropsychology. Drs. Tazeau and Karel have been on the forefront of APA task forces and committees developing guidelines to address these professional issues for the care of older adults. Dr. Vacha-Haase is a supervising psychologist and research mentor at a university doctoral program in counseling psychology who also maintains a practice with older adults, thereby reflecting the best features of a practitioner/scientist.

Unfortunately, due to space limitations, not all the important topics related to geropsychology competencies could be included in a volume this size. I note the absence of extended discussions of some gero-specific interventions such as reminiscence therapy for depression, end-of-life care for the terminally ill, bereavement therapy for complicated grief, and psychological treatments for those with mild cognitive problems.

In closing, I want to make due mention that all the senior authors of this volume have been significant in the development of applied geropsychology either through teaching via authorship of seminal textbooks, through science via the publication of research that advances the scholarly understanding of assessment and interventions with older adults, or through practice with day-to-day clinical work with older adults. It has been a pleasure to edit this volume knowing that readers will share in their collective wisdom.

Victor Molinari, PhD, ABPP

References

Hinrichsen, G. A., Zeiss, A. M., Karel, M. J., & Molinari, V. A. (2010). Competency-based training in doctoral internship and postdoctoral fellowships. *Training and Education in Professional Psychology, 4*(2), 91–98.

Karel, M. J., Knight, B. G., Duffy, M., Hinrichsen, G. A., & Zeiss, A. M. (2010). Attitude, knowledge, and skill competencies for practice in professional geropsychology: Implications for training and building a geropsychology workforce. *Training and Education in Professional Psychology, 4*(2), 75–84.

Knight, B. G., Karel, M. J., Hinrichsen, G. A., Qualls, S. H., & Duffy, M. (2009). Pikes Peak model for training in professional geropsychology. *American Psychologist, 64*(3), 205–214.

PART I

Knowledge Competencies

ONE

Professional Identification

Victor Molinari

The History of Geropsychology

The development of professional geropsychology as a discipline was largely a post–World War II phenomenon. Most of the early leaders in the field were researchers who were members of Division 20, Adult Development and Aging, of the American Psychological Association (APA). From its inception in 1946 (originally the first APA expansion division was called Division on Maturity and Old Age), Division 20 was not only the birthplace but also for a long time the only home for psychologists interested in older adults (Birren & Stine-Morrow, 1996). These formative years focused on aging as a research phenomenon and saw a dramatic increase in the understanding of normal and abnormal psychological aging. The 1970s saw the publication of a number of fairly extensive compendiums of the expanding knowledge base such as *The Psychology of Adult Development and Aging* (Eisdorfer & Lawton, 1973), *The Handbook of the Psychology of Aging* (Birren & Schaie, 1977), and *Aging in the 1980's* (Poon, 1980) that compiled the latest research findings in the basic psychology of aging. Much of this early research focused on the differences in cognitive performance between older and younger adults, but some of this work had a more applied interest and discussed intervention and caregiver issues (Storandt, 1983). Although the scholarly knowledge base of geropsychology continued to outpace professional developments for sometime to come, in the 1970s and 1980s intrepid clinically trained psychologists had already begun to put this burgeoning knowledge to practical use by "specializing" in working with older adults. Doyle Gentry's *Geropsychology: A Model of Training and Clinical Service* (1977), Storandt, Siegler and Elias's (1978) edited volume

The Clinical Psychology of Aging, Steve Zarit's *Aging and Mental Disorders* (1980), Richard Hussian's *Geriatric Psychology: A Behavioral Perspective* (1981), Bob Knight's *Psychotherapy with Older Adults* (1986), and Teri and Lewinsohn's *Geropsychological Assessment and Treatment* (1986) had a large impact on the practice community, demonstrating that the field of clinical geropsychology was mature enough to generate volumes showcasing the interest in and unique elements of conducting mental health assessment and treatment with older adults and their families.

In 1981 the first conference on Training Psychologists for Work in Aging took place in Boulder, Colorado. Dubbed the "Older Boulder" Conference, this meeting emphasized the identification of the core corpus of geropsychology knowledge, the development of training curricula, and the recruitment of new students to the field. The attendees advanced many prescient recommendations, especially encouraging the incorporation of aging content into psychology training curricula, the exposure to both healthy and frail older adults, the need for a multidisciplinary approach to treat older clients, and the use of varied models for different training levels including continuing education for licensed psychologists who desired additional skills in working with older adults (Knight, Santos, Teri & Lawton, 1995). Unfortunately, by and large these recommendations were not followed because at this time psychologists could not be reimbursed under Medicare for services to older adults, with the practice aspects of working with this population stifled by the broad health care system and the budget cutbacks of the 1980s (Hinrichsen & Zweig, 2005; Knight, Santos, Teri, & Lawton, 1995). Nevertheless, one major derivative of this conference was the launching in 1986 of APA's first aging-related journal, *Psychology and Aging*.

Happily, the professional climate dramatically changed in 1989 when the Omnibus Budget Reconciliation Act (OBRA) permitted Medicare to directly compensate licensed psychologists for supplying mental health services to older patients in a variety of settings (Norris, Molinari, & Rosowsky, 1998). Spurred by this ruling, professional geropsychology began to realize that it needed to align itself as much with clinical practice (i.e., Division 12, then called the Division of Clinical Psychology) as with the Division 20 scientific side for it to mature as an applied discipline. An initial attempt to establish a Division 12 geropsychology section in the early 1980s failed due to a perceived lack of sufficient numbers of geropsychologists and a professional ambience that was not yet ripe. However, following a second national conference in 1992, "Clinical Training in Psychology: Improving Services for Older Adults" (Knight et al., 1995) that was cosponsored by APA and the National Institute of Mental Health (NIMH), leaders in the field finally were able to forge a new section of Division 12 (Section 2: Clinical Geropsychology) in 1993. The formation of this section of professional psychologists interested in geropsychology was in recognition of the daunting demographics of aging, the reimbursement of psychologists under Medicare/Medicaid allowing more psychologists working in geriatric settings to earn an adequate living, and the growing number of internships (especially Veterans Administration programs due to the aging of World War II, Korean Conflict, and more recently Vietnam War veterans) offering training rotations with older adults. The division's first president was Mick Smyer, and its mission was "to support and to encourage the evolution and development of the subspecialty of clinical geropsychology in both its scientific and professional aspects" (Society of Clinical Geropsychology Web site, http://geropsych.org/, accessed 10/20/08).

In these early years, Division 12, Section 2 (today called the Society of Clinical Geropsychology) launched a variety of initiatives. With its LISTSERV, newsletter, and sponsorship of APA symposia and workshops at the American Psychological Association and Gerontological Society Association conventions, it allowed its members to consolidate an identity for themselves as "card-carrying" geropsychologists who conduct aging research, provide geriatric training, and assess and treat older adult clients. It also grappled with the question of what unique portfolio of knowledge and skills specifically distinguishes geropsychologists from other psychologists employed in settings where older adults are served.

As the clinical practice arena progressed due to improved reimbursement, one group of high-need frail older adults residing in long-term care settings was targeted because they have traditionally received "short shrift" regarding their mental health and quality of life needs. For this reason, many of the members of the Society of Clinical Geropsychology joined an informal APA-affiliated group, Psychologists in Long Term Care (PLTC), an organization founded by Joyce Parr in 1981 and nurtured by Michael Duffy in the mid-1980s. PLTC's mission has been to provide high-quality psychological services in long-term care settings such as nursing homes and assisted living facilities (www.pltcweb.org). Encouraged by the seminal research of Lawton (1975) in planning optimal living environments for older adults, and Camp et al. (1993), Burgio (1996), and Cohen-Mansfield (2001) in documenting the effectiveness of interventions in nursing home settings, PLTC targets very old adults who need specialized psychological assistance to address their day-to-day needs. Its 200 active members provide clinical services, conduct research, and do training to improve the lives of frail older adults. They network with each other to understand the labyrinth of regulatory mechanisms that undergirds our system of long-term care. In 1998, PLTC members published the *Standards for Psychological Services in Long Term Care Facilities* to promote the ethical administration of geriatric mental health care by psychologists (Lichtenberg et al., 1998). They have been particularly active in the advocacy arena, promoting mental health parity and the need for fair reimbursement of psychological assessment and treatment rendered in nursing homes and assisted-living facilities.

Given that APA was developing new mechanisms for subfield recognition during the early 1990s, some geropsychologists made preliminary forays to advance clinical geropsychology within APA by defining the specific parameters of applied geropsychology. It became imperative for geropsychology to distinguish itself from the related fields of neuropsychology, rehabilitation psychology, and health psychology. What skills are necessary for one to be considered a geropsychologist, and how much and what types of training are necessary for students to gain these skills? The second national conference, "Clinical Training in Psychology: Improving Services for Older Adults" (Knight et al., 1995), held in 1992, focused on training themes vis-à-vis clinical service needs and inspired discussions of issues regarding the certification of competence. A major accomplishment was in the delineation of a Three E model of training that describes what all clinical psychologists should receive (Exposure to working with older adults), what those who might be certified as being proficient should be provided (Experience with a variety of older adults in a variety of settings), and finally what those who consider themselves specialists should possess (Expertise in knowledge and skills across a variety of different aging-related practice areas) (Hinrichsen & Zweig, 2005).

Emanating from this conference was a debate about the pros and cons of the credentialing of geropsychologists who met certain criteria. This was posited to have the benefit of promoting the public interest by helping to assure that older clients were served by those who had attained at least minimum standards, by guiding training via mapping the knowledge and skills necessary for one to be labeled as a geropsychologist, by attracting others to the field with an official imprimatur, by marketing of services to managed care companies, and by defining a specific group of practitioners who could be considered expert resources within APA to provide clinical geropsychology with an identity as a specific field (Niederehe, Gatz, Taylor, & Teri, 1995). Credentialing became viewed as a process to offer up-to-date educational experiences and to support those interested in working with older people to meet training standards so as to provide optimal care.

Also derivative from this second training in aging conference was a project launched as a joint venture by Division 12, Section 2, and Division 20 (spearheaded by George Niederehe and Linda Teri) to develop and promulgate guidelines for the practice of geropsychology. It came to be understood that the term *geropsychology* needed to have official APA status for the discipline to move forward (Niederehe et al., 1995). In 1997, the Interdivisional Task Force on Qualifications for Practice in Clinical and Applied Geropsychology submitted a request to APA's Committee for the Recognition of Specialties and Proficiencies in Psychology that it recognize geropsychology as a proficiency area, and in 1998 this request was ultimately approved by the Council of Representatives (Norman, Ishler, Ashcraft, & Patterson, 2000). Another product of this Task Force (and years of toil) was approval by the Council of Representatives and publication of *Guidelines for Psychological Practice with Older Adults* (American Psychological Association, 2004). This became the first formal document identifying 20 guidelines reflecting the attitudes; general knowledge about adult development, aging, and older adults; clinical issues; assessment, intervention, consultation, and other service provision; and education for psychologists working clinically with older adults.

The Committee on Aging (CONA)

Although the Society of Clinical Geropsychology and PLTC represented giant steps forward for the advancement of our discipline by mobilizing its members, and proficiency status yielded an organizational cachet, there was also a recognition in the 1990s that geropsychology needed to have a permanent voice within the APA hierarchy to be able to have a greater impact on research, training, and practice policy. The visibility of geropsychology issues was heightened when Norm Abeles became president of APA in 1997. Exhibiting expertise in both geropsychology and neuropsychology, Dr. Abeles was acutely aware of the needs of practicing geropsychologists. He convened a task force that published a brochure "What Practitioners Should Know about Working with Older Adults" (American Psychological Association Working Group on the Older Adult, 1997, 1998), and assembled a second task force to develop a set of guidelines for dementia assessment. A mini-convention on aging was held at the annual APA meeting, and the proceedings were published as a volume by the APA Press (Qualls & Abeles, 2000). Perhaps of most importance, culminating follow-up efforts to the 1992 training conference, which had led to the establishment of the APA Ad Hoc Committee on Issues of the Older Adult

(Powell Lawton, chair), Dr. Abeles was able to push through pending "legislation" to establish a standing Committee on Aging (CONA). CONA is housed within the Office on Aging in the Public Interest Directorate and has become the institutional home for geropsychology within APA governance. Its mission is "to advance psychology as a science and profession and as a means of promoting human welfare by ensuring that older adults, especially the growing numbers of older women and minorities, receive the attention of the Association" (CONA Web site www. apa.org/pi/aging/cona01.html, accessed 10/18/08). Under the steady, guiding hand of Debbie DiGilio, director of APA's Office on Aging, CONA has gradually asserted itself as the body that pushes forward geropsychology initiatives that foster aging within APA by sponsoring workshops, drafting resolutions, and developing initiatives in collaboration with other APA directorates. Some recent projects include handbooks for lawyers and judges on assessment of capacity in older adults (co-written by the American Bar Association's Commission on Law and Aging 2005, 2006), a brochure describing what psychologists can do to help clients secure a fulfilling old age (APA, 2005), and a report addressing the challenges of providing interdisciplinary health care to older adults (APA, 2008). Working with the Society of Clinical Geropsychology and Division 20, CONA has also been supportive of efforts to refine the definition of clinical geropsychology.

Recent Developments in Geropsychology

The turn of this century has validated the predictions of demographers about the aging of the population, promoting a period of professional fervor and scientific scrutiny for geropsychologists. Clinical interventions have been increasingly subjected to the rigors of controlled research. Gatz et al. (1998) published an influential article documenting the empirical support for a number of psychological treatments for older adults, and more recently Scogin (2007) coordinated a series of articles on "evidence-based treatment for older adults" in a special issue of *Psychology and Aging*. With these developments has come an acknowledgment that much more needs to be accomplished professionally for geropsychologists to achieve status commensurate with the enhanced importance of mental health issues of older adults. Despite efforts to augment the numbers of psychologists providing services to older adults, there are perhaps only 700 self-identified geropsychologists in the field (Gatz, Karel, & Wolkenstein, 1991), an estimate that has remained constant over the years. In a survey of 1,227 psychologist practitioners, it was found that even though 70% of the respondents provided limited services to older adults, projected demand far outstripped supply (Qualls, Segal, Norman, Niederehe, & Gallagher-Thompson, 2002). Furthermore, although geropsychology internship rotations and postdoctoral fellowships are definitely increasing (Hinrichsen, Myers, & Stewart, 2000), the number of graduate programs offering a track or concentration in geropsychology clinical programs remains woefully low and not commensurate with the ever-rising need.

In 2004, a setback occurred when geropsychology's status as a proficiency came up for its required periodic review. APA's Committee for the Recognition of Specialties and Proficiencies in Psychology (CRSSP) rejected the application for recognition of geropsychology as a new specialty area, citing not enough well-developed training models as a main reason for geropsychology to maintain proficiency status. This decision sparked an introspective process within the field that prompted geropsychologists to recognize that we are at a turning point and must become better organized to advance professionally. Although recently an entire issue of the journal *Gerontology and Geriatrics Education* had been devoted to geropsychology at the doctoral, internship, postdoctoral, and Continuing Education (CE) levels (cf. Hinrichsen & Zweig, 2005), the leaders in geropsychology conceded the necessity to mobilize the practice, clinical research, and public policy sectors of the field for a national conference to review all aspects of geropsychology as a profession. There was a special recognition that although training models at all levels are needed, more developed CE opportunities are paramount to assure that high-quality services are delivered to older adults, many of whom are being treated by psychologists who through no fault of their own were not trained in geropsychology but are now increasingly faced with managing the complex biopsychosocial issues of older adults in their practices. The major questions on the minds of geropsychologists were how to classify the unique elements of who we are, and how to recognize what is essential about what we know.

After a lengthy planning process, in June 2006 the National Conference on Training in Professional Geropsychology (referred to as the Pikes Peak conference hereafter in this volume) was held in Colorado Springs, the home of the first APA-approved doctoral program in clinical geropsychology at the University of Colorado at Colorado Springs (UCCS). Organized by Bob Knight at the University of Southern California, Michele Karel of the Boston Veterans Administration, and Sara Qualls of UCCS, the conference included representatives from all the relevant geropsychology and general psychology stakeholders. It was short on presentations but long on work groups that performed the painstaking task of forging a very detailed map of the attitudes, knowledge, and skills involved in the core competencies needed for functioning as a geropsychologist. Although all participants understood that major progress has been made in professional geropsychology over the last decades, it was clear that a comprehensive plan was necessary. A "white paper" was written to help organize the knowledge in the field and point to directions for future growth (Karel, 2008a). A manuscript derived from the Pikes Peak conference was recently published in the *American Psychologist* (Knight, Karel, Hinrichsen, Qualls, & Duffy, 2009), and a series of articles derived from this conference have been have been accepted for publication in the APA journal *Training and Education in Professional Psychology* (Hinrichsen, Zeiss, Karel, & Molinari, 2010; Karel et al., 2010). A by-product of this feverish activity (and indeed of all the aforementioned geropsychology guidelines and training conferences) can be seen in the chapters of this present volume for which the Pikes Peak conference proceedings served as a model. (Please also see in this volume the chapter by Qualls, "The field of geropsychology" regarding how the Pikes Peak conference related to historical developments in geropsychology.)

The Pikes Peak conference also provided a catalyst for the formation of the Council of Geropsychology Training Programs (CoPGTP; www.usc.edu/programs/cpgtp) designed to further the work of this conference. "CoPGTP is committed to the promotion of excellence in training in professional geropsychology and to supporting the development of high quality training programs in professional geropsychology at the graduate school, internship, postdoctoral fellowship, and post-licensure levels of training" (Web site accessed10/14/08). CoPGTP now has nine doctoral programs and 10 internship training site members. A CoPGTP task force has developed and is now validating an instrument that will assist supervisors and supervisees in identifying areas of professional growth in geropsychology by yoking assessment items to specific knowledge and skill competencies.

Fulfilling the professional mission of geropsychology has been facilitated by the volume of excellent publications in geriatric mental health care over the last decade. For basic reading in applied geropsychology, Smyer and Qualls' (1999) *Aging and Mental Health* (now currently in its second edition; Segal, Qualls, & Smyer, in press) and Whitboune's (2001) *Psychopathology in Later Adulthood* are excellent places to start. Michael Duffy's (1999) *Handbook of Counseling and Psychotherapy with Older Adults* is a compendium of current thinking in the treatment of older adults. Lichtenberg's (1999; in press) *Handbook of Assessment in Clinical Gerontology* presents a broad state of the art look at clinical assessment with older adults. Hyer and Intrieri's (2006) *Geropsychological Interventions in Long Term Care* is a fine introduction to the provision of psychological treatment in long-term care settings. To keep professionals current with practitioner-relevant news in geropsychology, Hartman-Stein publishes a column in the *National Psychologist.*

Conclusions

Geropsychology once again has been put forward to be considered as an APA specialty, and the psychology aging community anxiously awaits this decision. The hope is that achievement of specialty status will serve as a vehicle for APA members to recognize that geropsychology is an exciting growth field. There are still far too few geropsychologists to provide optimal mental health services even to the neediest older adults, and we must publicize to the APA hierarchy and membership the tremendous potential of aging specialists to "train the trainers" to fulfill these needs. There also have been preliminary discussions with the American Board of Professional Psychology (ABPP) to develop board certification for geropsychology as a further designation that ours is a field whose time has come. The lengthy process and investment of resources that cultivating this type of certification requires will test the mettle of geropsychology, but one way or the other it will further define who we are and determine our direction in terms of the professionalization of the field.

Although geropsychology's growth as a discipline has been steady and the applied research and professional achievements impressive, we have a long road ahead to achieve our ultimate goals. First, the knowledge base regarding interventions with older adults must continue to expand to undergird the service activities of clinical geropsychologists. Interventions must be based on the available empirical evidence tempered by clinical realities and experiential wisdom gained by the often multifaceted but always rewarding process of working with older adult clients.

Second, competencies of professional geropsychologists must be further delineated. How do we assess for competencies at the varied exposure, experience, and expertise levels? The word needs to be disseminated that there is a significant corpus of unique attitudes, knowledge, and skills that geropsychologists bring to bear on the clinical situation that are more likely to render positive outcomes for their older patients.

Third, based on the decision that APA renders regarding specialty status, the geropsychology leadership will proceed accordingly and continue its push for organizational recognition.

Fourth, after APA specialty status is achieved, we will need to determine whether to commit time and energy to an ABPP application. This investment will be a large one but may pay off in dividends by having a major body outside of APA provide affirmation of our status by a rigorous examination of competencies and a credentialing process that is acknowledged nationally.

Fifth, given the aging demographics of the population, we must infuse knowledge of geriatric mental health throughout all professional psychology programs. It is imperative to expose graduate students as early as possible to material on aging in their coursework, and to experiences with older adults in practica supervised by aging-savvy psychologists. It's no longer acceptable for geriatrics to be relegated to the final chapters of developmental textbooks or for trainees' clinical work with older adults to be supervised by a psychologist who is not proficient in geropsychology.

Sixth, regarding APA activities, CONA, the Society of Clinical Geropsychology, and Division 20 must continue to endorse doctoral programs with geropsychology concentrations; to promote internships with "major" rotations with older adults supervised by specialists in geropsychology; to develop specific life-span training criteria that must be met for all APA-approved graduate, internship, and postdoctoral generalist programs; and to provide continuing education workshops, symposia, papers, and posters on applied geropsychology at the annual convention.

Seventh, special sections of varied APA divisions that work with older adults should be cultivated and linked together. Merla Arnold, past chair of CONA has been the linchpin for such an initiative and has developed a special aging section within Division 17 (Counseling Psychology). Relatedly, we must recognize that as clinical geropsychology grows and develops, there will be natural sub-areas within this field such as long-term care, gerontological neuropsychology, gerontological rehabilitation, multicultural gerontology, and psychologists providing services to dying patients and their families. It will be a challenge for the field to continue to nurture integrative ties among these related areas and to avoid the divisive splits that could impede the necessary cross-fertilization so vital for the growth of geropsychology.

Eighth, likewise, state associations should be broached regarding forming special geriatric sections and be encouraged to offer professional geropsychology training workshops to their members.

Ninth, APA's Practice, Research, Education and Public Interest Directorates must be implored to coordinate their varied aging initiatives so that aging can be 'promoted' to its members.

And tenth, geriatric mental health advocacy initiatives at the local, state, and national levels must be coordinated with those of varied psychological and mental health groups. Lobbying must be intensified and earmarked for greater funding of aging research at NIMH and National Institute of Aging, for more programs targeting geropsychology training (e.g., Health Resources Services Administration-sponsored Geropsychology Graduate Psychology Training), and for fair reimbursement procedures under Medicare, Medicaid, and managed care systems. As one example, CONA has developed strong ties with the National Coalition of Mental Health and Aging and is assisting with endeavors to educate legislators about the need for geriatric mental health.

Professional geropsychology has had a relatively short history but appears poised for a long and bright future. Professional geropsychologists must be competent as clinical psychologists and proficient as geriatric mental health experts as well. Building the science with rigorous quantitative and qualitative research on interventions in older adults and enhancing teaching via supervision and mentoring of students at all levels will promote the delineation of competencies and will maintain our professional growth as scientist practitioners in this exciting area. The demographics beckon us to demarcate our identity and to continue to evolve as geropsychologists in the service of our rapidly aging population.

TWO

The Field of Geropsychology

Sara Honn Qualls

The development of competencies in geropsychology represents another key step in the maturation of the professional practice of psychology with older adults. The science and practice of psychology related to aging expanded rapidly in the second half of the 20th century, marking several other key steps of maturation, all of which readied the field to define the competencies needed to practice in this discipline. This chapter identifies the discipline of geropsychology (The Psychology of Aging) as a distinct discipline in research and practice, articulates central tenets of the theoretical framework, and explores overlaps with related disciplines.

What Is Geropsychology?

Geropsychology encompasses research and practice related to aging that arises within the field of psychology. In contrast, gerontology is a multidisciplinary field that addresses all aspects of aging, including but not limited to psychology. The term *geropsychology* is the shorter term that is gaining in common usage in recent decades among health professionals and in library reference materials (Tuleya, 2007). Publications within the American Psychological Association (APA) define geropsychology as the "specialized field of psychology concerned with the psychological and behavioral aspects of aging" (Tuleya, 2007). This term was adopted by the APA to describe the field in 2006 and has been applied retrospectively as a keyword within the APA publication databases.

The field of geropsychology has emerged due to strong population demands that result from the aging of the population. Despite the demographic shifts and evidence of increasing utilization of mental health services by older adults (Robb, Haley, Becker, Polivka, & Chwa, 2003), the workforce in the field is small. A survey of APA members who self-identified as practitioners found that fewer than 4% of them identified their work as primarily focused on older adults (Qualls, Segal, Norman, Niederehe, & Gallagher-Thompson, 2002). Psychology joins other health disciplines that are all experiencing the problem of having a training pipeline that is far too small to meet the needs of the aging population (Halpain, Harris, McClure, Jeste, 1999; Institute of Medicine, 2008).

Professional geropsychology refers to clinical, counseling, or other applied work with older adults that draws upon the field of psychology to understand or intervene in human behavior. With expertise in working with older adults' mental and behavioral health problems, geropsychologists draw from knowledge and skills in related subdisciplines such as health psychology, neuropsychology, rehabilitation psychology, and end-of-life care. For example, the increased probability of chronic illness in older adults means that patients or clients of geropsychologists will benefit from assistance in self-management of illness, for which health psychology has valuable models. However, illness is not the sole or even primary focus of work with older adults, so health psychologists cannot fill the entire niche covered by geropsychology. Similarly, geropsychologists have experience in neuropsychology in order to address cognitive impairments due to age-related diseases. Although most geropsychologists lack the expertise to conduct neuropsychological evaluations, they are knowledgeable consumers of technical reports that psychologists working with other adult populations would rarely encounter. In essence, geropsychologists must have working knowledge from each of these subdisciplines to effectively address the holistic well-being of older adults. Consistent with ethical standards, geropsychologists provide only those services for which they have expertise and refer clients to experts for specialty services that extend beyond their competency level.

The work of professional geropsychologists includes consultation, direct services, environmental interventions, and community interventions. Because older adults become more dependent on the supports available in their environments, geropsychologists have a key role to play in assisting older adults, their families, and their communities with interventions that are not commonly part of psychologists' work with younger adults. For example, geropsychologists must be familiar with issues of environmental design and adaptive technologies. Community interventions might include efforts to improve public health (e.g., depression screenings).

Geropsychology has embraced integrative care models that place psychological services into settings where older adults seek services, such as primary care or senior services agencies (APA, 2008).

References to aging as a distinct phase of the life span require some explanation of the point at which the reference applies to individuals. In other words, what is the magic age when aging is the correct descriptor for one's work? Although public policies in the United States have targeted age 65 as the focal point for many entitlement policies (e.g., Medicare and Social Security), no clear chronological marker is used in geropsychology. This particular age was selected almost 80 years ago for use in the policies of one particular country. No specific marker was associated with it that dictated the selection of that particular age. Indeed, aging processes do not map well onto particular ages. Instead, aging is conceptualized as a process that occurs throughout the life span, with varied trajectories of gain and loss in particular domains of functioning (Baltes & Baltes, 1990). Identifying variations across populations in the timing of gains and losses represents a significant portion of the scientific work of geropsychologists.

The profession organizes aging-related work within the context of adult development so as to provide a broader context for understanding human behavior. For example, the primary organizational home for aging within APA is Division 20, the Adult Development and Aging division. Course titles in university curricula that are labeled the Psychology of Aging use textbooks that are entitled *Adult Development and Aging* (e.g., Cavanaugh & Blanchard-Fields, 2006). Even the earliest longitudinal studies of aging examined adults who were in late midlife and older (Neugarten, 1973).

The ultimate goal of geropsychology is to apply scientific findings about psychological aging to improve the lives of older adults. Scientific studies of aging investigate age-related changes using sophisticated research methods that allow scientists to explain those changes. Geropsychologists work to distinguish between normal changes associated with age from those that are driven by age-related diseases. Normal aging and age-related diseases are presumed to co-occur at times in older adults, challenging efforts to distinguish them. Some older adults have no pathological conditions and are simply viewed by geropsychologists as adults at a different stage in the life span who are experiencing the same processes as other adults. Although often associated with illnesses such as dementias, geropsychology is a far broader discipline requiring a rich understanding of the full range of human behavior.

Geropsychology operates within a biopsychosocial framework that emphasizes the rich sources of variability in human behavior that arise from biological, psychological, and social factors. Furthermore, factors within each of the three categories demonstrate complex interrelationships that directly or indirectly influence any outcome of interest in older adults. Thus, all domains of psychology overlap with geropsychology when particular behavioral outcomes are examined.

Life-Span Developmental Psychology

Grounded in life-span developmental theory, geropsychology shares major tenets of the developmental paradigm. The central construct of all developmental paradigms is that change occurs across the life span, offering opportunities for adaptation at all ages, including late life. The primacy of change processes leads geropsychologists to focus on intraindividual changes as well as interindividual differences at particular moments in time. Of particular interest are interindividual differences in intraindividual change. Older adults are highly heterogeneous, reflecting lifetimes of within-individual change trajectories. Geropsychologists respect the diversity among older adults and recognize the varied developmental pathways by which older adults achieved this variation.

Life-span developmental psychological theories recognize that development occurs in both continuous and discontinuous processes that are multidirectional and multidimensional (Baltes, Lindenberger, & Staudinger, 2006). Some developmental changes are the culmination of steady, consistent changes over time. Others appear to be qualitative shifts in organizational complexity, adaptive processes, or capabilities. All developmental periods from childhood to advanced old age are characterized by both gains and losses, with variable patterns evident across domains of functioning. The multidimensionality of development acknowledges that gains in one domain may occur simultaneously with losses in another. Although the balance tilts toward proportionally greater losses than gains in old age, both gains and losses characterize development even in advanced old age. Plasticity refers to the ability to adapt to characteristics of specific contexts (Lerner, 1984).

Geropsychologists rely on developmental theories to explain the interplay of person-environment interaction (Bronfenbrenner & Morris, 2006). The ecology of human development examines the impact of characteristics of the proximal environments, the mid-level environment in which proximal systems interact, and the macro-environmental factors that influence the broader cultural and biological systems in which humans live (Bronfenbrenner & Morris, 2006). Older adults are viewed by geropsychologists as adaptive in response to characteristics of each level of the environment.

Life events offer one lens for studying developmental processes across the life span. Developmental theory distinguishes between events that are structured by culture to occur at particular ages (age-graded), events that occur as a product of history (history-graded), and events that are non-normative. All three categories are experienced across the life span, although later life is more heavily influenced by non-normative events than other age periods. Geropsychologists trace the influence of life events on the person and the environment, and the adaptive processes used by individuals in particular environments.

The fact that human behavior is multidimensional and embedded in multiple levels of environmental contexts that change over time requires geropsychologists to use multidisciplinary, longitudinal approaches to scientific endeavors as well as applied work. Neither researchers nor practitioners can work in isolation from other disciplines because the aging processes that are the focus of their work lead to cross disciplinary inquiry. For clinicians, teams are the basic unit of functioning, even if the teams are virtual rather than interactive. Researchers must collaborate to examine the interplay of factors that influence aging processes. Furthermore, the measurement and analysis of behavior over time is fundamental to the study of aging processes (Schaie, 1983). Addressing contextual variables across layers of the human ecology adds richness and complexity to research designs and professional practice.

The Pikes Peak Model of Training in Professional Geropsychology

The history of geropsychology provides a rich and useful backdrop for understanding the principles adopted within the Pikes Peak Model of Training in Professional Geropsychology (Knight, Karel, Hinrichsen, Qualls, & Duffy, 2009). The competencies in professional geropsychology practice that were articulated in the Pikes Peak Model followed the organization of other competencies models (Kaslow et al., 2007) around attitudes, knowledge, and skill. The model emphasizes the foundational role of attitudes and knowledge about aging in the implementation of clinical skills. Because ageism pervades our society with significant deleterious effects on the functioning of older people as well as others' responses to older adults, attitudinal training has particular importance (Levy, Zonderman, Slade, & Ferrucci, 2009). Respect for diversity within the aging population requires geropsychologists to understand the historical context within which a particular birth cohort lived, and the social influences of that historical context on persons varying in categories that afforded particular privileges in a particular time and place.

Geropsychologists must understand the differences between normative age-related change and pathologies, and, as aforementioned, this requires knowledge from areas including (but not limited to) health psychology, neuropsychology, rehabilitation psychology, and end-of-life issues. Knowledge of the science of psychology includes the substantial body of literature within life-span developmental psychology as well as the interaction of developmental processes with issues related to life events common in later life, illnesses and medications, family and social structures, and cognitive and physical changes associated with age. Developmental research offers some of the strongest empirical bases for professional practice that exist to date. Interventions are often a logical extension of descriptive and explanatory research that results in theoretical propositions about intervention. The knowledge base in these areas leads to informed assessment, case formulation, flexible treatments in a variety of settings with clients from diverse cultures, and consultation with other disciplines.

The distinctive aspects of assessment and treatment skills with older adults also are rooted in a scientific knowledge base. Professional practice with older adults requires a rich knowledge of the broader assessment and intervention literature because work with older adults is in many ways more similar to, than different from, work with other adults (Knight, 2004). However, knowledge of the distinct assessment and intervention literatures are also critical to geropsychologists (Duffy, 1999; Lichtenberg, 1999; in press). Outcome and efficacy research on psychopathology treatment in older populations has a distinct knowledge base, for example (Scogin, 2007). Similarly, many distinctive assessment tools support professional practice with older adults, including, for example, particular tools to differentiate dementia from depression. Distinctive norms are also critically important, including norms that are age-specific, and often population-specific (Manly, 2006).

In sum, the Pikes Peak Model grounds professional practice skills in the attitudes and knowledge of the profession broadly, as well as the distinctive aspects of professional work with older adults.

Conclusion

Following the rapid aging of society in the 20th century, geropsychology emerged as a distinct discipline in which the competencies for professional practice are grounded. The science of geropsychology is based in life span developmental psychology but draws on many related fields (e.g., health psychology, cognitive, environmental, and neuropsychology). Professional geropsychology includes practice by counselors, clinicians, and consultants among others for whom the biopsychosocial framework is critical to capture the complexity of changes in later life. Professional geropsychology competencies thus represent the expertise of a distinct field as the foundation for attitudes, knowledge, and skills of effective practice.

THREE

Conceptual and Scientific Foundations

Susan Krauss Whitbourne and Lauren A. Zeranski

This chapter is meant to provide a comprehensive overview of the aging process, including descriptions of the physical, psychological, social, and environmental challenges that can accompany later life. The processes described in this chapter are associated with normative aging. Nevertheless, it is important to recognize the great diversity in this age group, an understanding critical to an informed geropsychological practice.

The Biopsychosocial Perspective

Throughout this chapter, aging is viewed from the biopsychosocial perspective, which proposes that development is a complex interaction of biological, psychological, and social processes. In later life, biological processes associated with the passage of time include those that involve deleterious changes in the body's structures and functions, but they can also include adaptations involving brain plasticity and compensation through physiological and behavioral interventions. The psychological aspect of change in later life includes a slowing of processing speed and decreased working memory function but also the improvement or maintenance of abilities through education and experience. Social context is the third component of the biopsychosocial model and reflects changes in the individual's position within the social structure, including retirement and alterations in support networks.

The biopsychosocial model therefore takes a multidimensional approach to aging and also a multidirectional one, incorporating both loss and compensation (Baltes & Graf, 1996).

Although many changes in later life represent significant adaptational challenges, the majority of older adults are able to cope successfully with age-related changes and maintain their resilience in the face of stressful life events. In this chapter, the biopsychosocial model will be examined in the context of major age-related changes in later life with a focus on healthy outcomes and implications for clinical treatment. Because older adults are a highly diverse group (Nelson & Dannefer, 1992), geropsychologists should understand how the effects of these changes manifest themselves in normal aging in order to identify pathological presentations and responses.

Diversity in Aging

Before specific age-related changes are examined, it is important to challenge the myth that individuality fades as the aging process takes its toll on physical and psychological functioning. As people within a given cohort age, life paths become increasingly divergent from one another due to the variety of experiences they have in terms of health, education, career, family, and involvement in the larger community. Each individual's personal history moves in more idiosyncratic directions with each passing day, year, and decade of life.

Because of the wide diversity within the aging population, it is even possible to find older adults whose performance on a given measure is superior to that of younger people. An older adult who exercises and remains active may very well be quicker, stronger, and mentally more adept than a sedentary or inactive younger person. An imaging study of age-adjusted brain volumes in the lateral prefrontal cortex, primary visual cortex, and hippocampus found that some individuals in their 70s and 80s appear similar to or higher than participants in their 20s (Hedden & Gabrieli, 2004). Professional geropsychologists are sensitive to differences among older adults and keep the great diversity of this population in mind when assessing and treating their clients.

Age Demarcations in Later Life

Traditionally, age 65 is considered the entry point for "old age." However, individuals close to age 65 face very different issues and challenges from those who are close to age 85 or beyond. Consequently, gerontologists conceptualize later life as consisting of three age ranges: young-old (65 to 74), old-old (75 to 84), and oldest-old (ages 85 and over). Although transitions between these ranges are more gradual than simply passing a birthday, it is understood that within a year or two of entering these periods some changes will become apparent that may lead to significant changes in functioning. As implied by the biopsychosocial model, there can also be great diversity within these age groupings. Individuals who fall within the young-old age bracket may be grandparents or retirees; conversely some of the oldest-old are without grandchildren or still working. The diversity of older individuals defies any simple characterizations based on age alone.

With increases in life expectancy and the growth of the over-65 population, limitations for even these three age groupings have been recognized. Centenarians, people over the age of 100, and super-centenarians, those over the age of 110, are the two newest age categories to be added to the divisions of the older adult population. In addition to living longer, the overall population will live healthier lives well into their 90s and beyond (Centers for Disease Control and Prevention, 2007).

Normal Aging Versus Disease

Further reinforcing the notion of variability in aging, gerontologists differentiate among normal, impaired, and optimal aging. Normal aging involves changes that occur universally. Impaired aging applies to changes associated with disease. Optimal aging, or "successful aging," describes the processes through which older individuals avoid negative changes that would otherwise occur with age. This minimization of such deleterious processes as atherosclerosis, hypertension, and bone loss is often accomplished through preventive and compensatory strategies like exercise, mental activity, and judicious use of medications. Practical as well as scientific reasons drive the need for these distinctions. Health care practitioners should recognize and treat a disease when it occurs rather than attribute it to the normal aging process. At the same time, older adults should be encouraged whenever possible to take advantage of preventive and compensatory strategies to maintain healthy functioning.

MIND-BODY INTERACTIONS: COPING MECHANISMS

With advancing age, individuals may feel that they are losing control over vital areas of functioning, from the body to the social environment. Therefore, coping and self-efficacy have held great interest for gerontological researchers.

The MacArthur Study of Adult Development, a large, national U.S. survey of almost 3,500 adults, showed that despite awareness of increasing constraints in their lives, adults 60 and older feel high levels of control in their lives and are able to view their resources and potential positively rather than focusing on losses (Plaut, Markus, & Lachman, 2003).

Because coping successfully with stressful situations enhances the individual's mood, improved physical health may also be an outcome of active coping. In one study of community dwelling, active, older adults, the ability to take charge of potentially stressful situations before they become problematic was found to result in fewer subsequent stresses (Fiksenbaum, Greenglass, & Eaton, 2006). The relationship between coping and health is also reciprocal; successful coping can be facilitated by good health and extensive social networks (Brennan, Schutte, & Moos, 2006). Resilience can also facilitate the coping process (Ong, Bergeman, Bisconti, & Wallace, 2006). The ability to overcome negative emotions and adapt to new situations allows older adults to maintain a positive mood even during periods of high stress.

Some discussions of coping in later life regard older adults as passive rather than active copers. However, it is important to recognize that older adults typically are not fatalists. Instead, older adults normally show initiative in managing their life course. At the heart of their coping efforts is a desire to maintain a feeling of independence, even if they have been forced to relinquish some of their actual independence due to changes in functional abilities (Duner & Nordstrom, 2005).

Ageism

One of the more significant social forces that confronts older adults is ageism, the set of beliefs, attitudes, social institutions, and acts that denigrates individuals or groups based on their chronological age. Ageism may be positive or negative: Older adults are seen as "cute" or "kindly" as well as "senile" or "cranky" (Kite & Wagner, 2002). Whether positive or negative, the effects of ageism can nevertheless render older adults "invisible." Disengagement theory is the now out-of-date proposal that older adults gradually withdraw from activities in preparation for death. When popular, the theory only reinforced ageist views of older adults and to the extent that it is still discussed today, continues to do so. Though prohibited by law, ageism also exists in the workplace, where it subtly can result in unfair treatment of older workers, such as harsher penalties for mistakes that would be forgiven if made by younger workers (Rupp, Vodanovich, & Crede, 2006). At the heart of ageism, according to researchers and theorists, is the fear of mortality: By their presence, the old remind younger people of the inevitability of their own mortality (Martens, Greenberg, Schimel, & Landau, 2004). Geropsychologists must be sensitive to any subtle ageist beliefs that they may hold and also be aware of how ageism affects their clients.

Brain and Cognitive Changes in Later Life

AGE-RELATED STRUCTURAL BRAIN CHANGES

Previous research relied on autopsy results, so the advent of magnetic resonance imaging (MRI) has produced a wealth of information on the effects of normal aging that previously had been unobtainable. MRI studies reveal the most pronounced effects of normal aging on the prefrontal cortex, the area of the brain most involved in planning and the encoding of information into long-term memory, although there are significant individual variations in these cortical changes (Hedden & Gabrieli, 2004). The hippocampus, the brain structure involved in memory consolidation, becomes smaller with increasing age in adulthood (Schiltz et al., 2006), although this decline is more pronounced in the brains of people with dementia. These findings have aided the understanding of the neurological bases for changes in memory and cognitive functions related to attention in adulthood (Townsend, Adamo, & Haist, 2006).

Aging is also associated with the development of white matter hyperintensities (WMH), areas of cell death that appear as dense white shadows on MRI. Due to the great variability of the older adult population, the association between age and WMH may also reflect the probable inclusion of participants with pathological brain changes. The relationship between WMH and cognitive performance has not been clearly established (Raz & Rodrigue, 2006). Just as the presence of imaging findings does not necessarily signify impaired cognition, the absence of findings does not equal a clean slate. Geropsychologists consider how age-related cognitive changes affect the subjective experience of older adults and how they may adversely affect mental health.

PROCESSING SPEED

Age-related brain changes may underlie changes in psychomotor speed, the amount of time needed to process a signal, prepare a response, and then execute that response (Madden, 2001). The theory of attentional resources and aging proposes that older adults are slower because they have less energy available for cognitive operations (Blanchet, Belleville, & Peretz, 2006). Alternatively, the inhibitory deficit hypothesis suggests that aging reduces the individual's ability to tune out irrelevant information (Hasher, Zachs & May, 1999).

Although older adults may process visual information more slowly, they may be equally as capable of remembering where an item was in a visual display. In one study, older adults were more efficient than young adults in remembering where an item had appeared on a display, signaling faster visual search capabilities (Kramer et al., 2006).

WORKING MEMORY

Working memory, the component of memory in which information is temporarily stored and manipulated, is particularly vulnerable to the effects of aging, presumably due to the above-mentioned loss of hippocampal volume. Because they process newly presented information less efficiently, older adults often cannot effectively encode and retrieve that information, ultimately affecting their long-term episodic memory (Wingfield & Kahana, 2002).

Although the vast majority of memory studies are cross-sectional and hence subject to cohort effects, longitudinal data are available to confirm this general pattern of memory decline (Davis, Trussell, & Klebe, 2001; Zelinski & Burnight, 1997). However, even in this area, compensation is an important process that can counter the effects of aging on memory; older adults increase their activation of the frontal lobes when processing information in memory, presumably to offset the losses they experience in the hippocampus (Persson et al., 2006).

INTELLIGENCE

Crystallized intelligence, or acquired knowledge, continues to increase throughout adulthood as the individual gains knowledge and experience. Fluid intelligence, the ability to develop and infer abstract relationships, begins to decline in early adulthood and becomes more pronounced in midlife. However, the decline in fluid intelligence can be mitigated by training. A multisite investigation of training effects on a U.S. sample of over 2,800 older adults has produced impressive data showing that training in fluid inductive reasoning significantly improved older adults' functional abilities, an effect that was maintained over the 5-year period of the investigation (Willis et al., 2006).

Contextual Changes in Later Adulthood

WORK AND RETIREMENT

Compared to other celebratory rituals in adulthood, such as college graduation, marriage, and the birth of children, retirement is more likely to carry ambivalent associations for the individual due to the changes it entails in daily life and connections that are potentially lost to the world of work.

Retirement satisfaction is related to resources like finances, health, and quality of marital relationships, such that the loss of one of these supports decreases satisfaction (Van Solinge & Henkens, 2008). Adjustment to retirement involves acceptance of the loss of occupation and resultant changes to income and self-esteem as well as the replacement of formal work with new activities considered meaningful and enjoyable. Successful adjustment to retirement is also related to feelings of personal control. Retirement adjustment is maximized when individuals exit the work role in an "on-time" fashion with ample preparation time (Gill et al., 2006). A minimum of 2 years of planning prior to early retirement is related to a positive retirement experience compared to a decision made 6 months or less prior to retirement (Hardy & Quadagno, 1995).

Similarly, the reason for retirement can impact the individual's well-being. Although retirement can be a voluntary decision, research has shown that approximately 20% to 30% of older adults in Western countries consider their retirement forced or involuntary (Van Solinge & Henkens, 2008). When retirement is suddenly mandated due to downsizing, individuals suffer from this perceived loss of control and consequently diminished well-being (Armstrong-Stassen, 2001; Kalimo, Taris, & Schaufeli, 2003). Financial status also plays an important role. Depressive symptoms become an increasingly likely outcome if the retiree lacks sufficient financial resources (Gallo et al., 2006).

Continuity theory (Atchley, 1989) proposes that retirement in and of itself is not the cause of depressive symptoms, loss of identity, or negative social role changes. Because they continue to identify with their former work role, retirees maintain their previous goals, patterns of activities, and relationships. It is the desirability of their current role that determines whether retirement will be associated with lowered satisfaction (Warr, Butcher, Robertson, & Callinan, 2004).

FAMILY LIFE AND CLOSE RELATIONSHIPS

Not surprisingly, parent-child relationships maintain their importance throughout life (Allen, Blieszner, & Roberto, 2000). For older adults, and particularly for women, these relationships can play a vital role in well-being (An & Cooney, 2006). For example, the quality of parent-child relationships is related to mental health outcomes such as loneliness and depression among aging parents (Koropeckyj-Cox, 2002).

Family life grows richer for many older adults when they become grandparents. At this point, they begin to enjoy the benefits of interactions with young children, but they are also able to avoid the more arduous tasks of parenthood. Unfortunately, not all grandparents are able to enjoy the benefits of their status due to distance or impaired relationships with their children, nor do all grandparents want to assume this role. Furthermore, increasingly grandparents are being asked to substitute for a parent who is not present in the home or whose job has extensive time commitments (U.S. Bureau of the Census, 2008).

Throughout the vicissitudes of marriage, divorce, remarriage, and widowhood, most adults actively strive to maintain daily gratifying interactions with others. Furthermore, for many adults, the feeling of being part of a close relationship or network of relationships is the most salient aspect of identity (Whitbourne, 1986). Whether this relationship is called "marriage," "family," "friendship," or "partnership" is not as important as the feeling that one is valued by others and has something to offer to improve the life of other people.

BEREAVEMENT

The death of a spouse is regarded as one of the most stressful events in life, and for many older adults, widowhood involves the loss of a relationship that may have lasted as long as 50 years or more. The survivor is faced with enormous readjustments in every aspect of life. Even when there is time to prepare, adjustment to widowhood is a difficult and painful process. Depressive symptoms may persist for several years after the loss (Wilcox, Evenson, Aragaki, Wassertheil-Smoller, Mouton, & Loevinger, 2003). Without remarriage, levels of well-being may not return to preexisting levels for as long as 8 years after the spouse's death (Lucas, Clark, Georgellis, & Diener, 2003).

Among the many ramifications of widowhood are loss of an attachment figure, interruption of the plans and hopes invested in the relationship, and construction of a new identity in accordance with the reality of being single (Field, Nichols, Holen, & Horowitz, 1999). People who are widowed are at higher risk of developing depression and anxiety disorders (Onrust & Cuijpers, 2006). They may experience phenomena such as sensing the presence, dreaming about, and having hallucinations or illusions of seeing or hearing the deceased (Lindstrom, 1995; LoConto, 1998). These manifestations of grief may persist for as long as 2.5 years (Ott & Lueger, 2002). Indeed the bereaved may continue to think about the spouse and even have "conversations" with the deceased on a weekly basis for as long as 35 years or more. Anniversary reactions may continue for over 50 years following the spouse's death (Carnelley, Wortman, Bolger, & Burke, 2006).

Individuals vary in their reactions to widowhood, and geropsychologists should be sensitive to the various types of grief reactions. Bonanno and collaborators (2002) identified five prominent patterns: common grief, chronic grief, chronic depression, improvement during bereavement, and resilience. The most common pattern is resilient grief, in which the bereaved person, perhaps remarkably, shows little or no distress following the loss. Personality also appears to play a role in affecting grief patterns. Those who showed the pattern of resilience were most accepting of death and were more likely to agree with the notion that the world is "just" (i.e., that people "get" what they "deserve"). High levels of interpersonal dependency were most likely to be associated with the chronic grief pattern. Adaptation to widowhood is influenced by prior levels of well-being. Those who are more vulnerable to widowhood's negative effects tend to be those who had lower well-being prior to their loss (Bennett, 2005).

Illnesses that involve marked physical and mental deterioration and place extensive burden on the caregivers also influence the bereaved's response to widowhood (Ferrario, Cardillo, Vicario, Balzarini, & Zotti, 2004). Following the spouse's death, relief from the pressures of caregiving can lead to alleviation of symptoms of depression and stress present during the spouse's dying months or years (Bonanno, Wortman, & Nesse, 2004).

Men seem particularly vulnerable to feelings of stress and depression after the death of their wives (Bennett, Smith, & Hughes, 2005; Stroebe, 2001). Widowers are at greater mortality risk within the first 6 months after bereavement than are widows, with a mortality rate estimated in one study to be 12 times higher for men than women for those over 75 years of age (Gallagher-Thompson, Futterman, Farberow, Thompson, & Peterson, 1993). Men are more likely to remarry, but women are more likely to form new friendships, particularly with neighbors (Lamme, Dykstra, & Broese Van Groenou, 1996). It is possible that social support plays a greater role in women's adaptation to widowhood, but for men (particularly current cohorts) a more relevant factor is the availability of practical support in performing household tasks (Gass, 1989).

Mood Disorders in Later Adulthood in Relation to Normal Aging

Depression is thought to be a natural part of the aging process due to the association of aging with loss. However, in contrast to stereotypes of older adults as depressed and dissatisfied with their lives, in reality data show that younger adults are more likely than their elders to suffer from a diagnosable mood disorder. Nevertheless, subthreshold depression remains an issue in the older adult population: between 8% and 20% of community-dwelling adults aged 65 and older are reported to experience depressive symptoms. Rates in primary care settings almost double that percentage (17% to 35%; Gurland, Cross, & Katz, 1996). Even though older adults may not meet the full diagnostic criteria for mood disorders, those who suffer from these symptoms are likely to be troubled by them for many years if left untreated (Beekman et al., 2002).

SYMPTOMS

Due to the high prevalence rate of subsyndromal depressive symptoms in older adults professional geropsychologists should be highly sensitive to mood symptoms in their clients. Complicating detection is the often atypical presentation of depressive symptoms in older adults, who are less likely to report some of the traditionally recognized depressive symptoms of dysphoria, guilt, low self-esteem, and suicidality. When they seek treatment, they are more likely to focus on somatic complaints such as pain and abdominal symptoms (Amore, Tagariello, Laterza, & Savoia, 2007) or on psychological symptoms that do not appear related to depression, such as anxiety, abnormalities in psychomotor functioning, cognitive dysfunction, and somatic or paranoid delusions (King & Markus, 2000).

RISK FACTORS

A phenomenon restricted to later adulthood is known as late-onset depression, a depression that first appears after the age of 60. Risk factors for late-onset depression include becoming a widow, having had less than a high school education, experiencing impairments in physical functioning, and being a heavy alcohol drinker (U.S. Department of Health and Human Services, 1999). Late-onset depression is more likely to be accompanied by psychotic symptoms including hypochondriacal and nihilistic delusions (Gournellis et al., 2001). Depression may also occur in conjunction with dementia, particularly in the early stages as individuals begin to come to grips with the implications of the disease for their future (Harwood, Sultzer, & Wheatley, 2000). It may also develop as part of the same underlying disease process as dementia (Palmer et al., 2007).

Several types of functional limitations can increase the older individual's risk of developing depression. These include sensory impairments (Lupsakko, Mantyjarvi, Kautiainen, & Sulkava, 2002), chronic illness

(Sneed, Kasen, & Cohen, 2006), disability (Oslin et al., 2002), and impaired memory and cognition (Gallo, Rebok, Tennsted, Wadley, & Horgas, 2003). Bereavement, isolation, and stressful life events can also serve as risk factors (Bruce, 2002). An inability to employ successful coping strategies to deal with late-life stressors can also increase the individual's risk of developing depression (Holahan, Moos, Holahan, Brennan, & Schutte, 2005).

Other predisposing risk factors that occur in later life and that may not be thought of as related to depressive symptoms include hip fracture (Lenze et al., 2007), tooth loss (Persson et al., 2003), and insufficient vitamin D in the diet (Wilkins, Sheline, Roe, Birge, & Morris, 2006). Physical disorders present in one's spouse, like urinary incontinence, may also contribute to depressive symptoms (Fultz et al., 2005).

Unfortunately, health care professionals are not well trained in recognizing these often atypical signs of depression in their older clients (Charney et al., 2003). Health care providers may consider depression a natural consequence of aging and pay less attention to its symptoms. Alternately, they may wish to avoid stigmatizing older clients by diagnosing them with a psychological disorder (Duberstein & Conwell, 2000). Misdiagnosis may also occur because the symptoms of mood disorders are seen in conjunction with a medical condition, leading either to failure to detect the mood disorder or misattribution of the symptoms (Delano-Wood & Abeles, 2005). The growing proportion of older adults in the population makes the understanding of geriatric mental health a public health imperative.

MORBIDITY AND MORTALITY

Over the long term, older adults who do not receive appropriate treatment for a mood disorder are at greater risk for developing a variety of impairments in physical and cognitive functioning (Chodosh, Kado, Seeman, & Karlamangla, 2007). Those older adults with more severe symptoms of depression and those whose depression is unremitting are more likely to experience higher rates of mortality over time (Geerlings, Beekman, Deeg, Twisk, & Van Tilburg, 2002). The relationship between depression and higher morbidity may be related to immune system dysfunction. Late-life depression is associated with inflammatory cytokines, signaling proteins that communicate with and activate immune cells, part of an overall elevated inflammatory response (Smith, Gunning-Dixon, Lotrich, Taylor, & Evans, 2007). These cytokines can eventually increase the risk of cardiovascular disease, osteoporosis, arthritis, type 2 diabetes, cancers, periodontal disease, frailty, and functional decline (Kiecolt-Glaser & Glaser, 2002).

GERIATRIC BIPOLAR DISORDER

Rates of bipolar disorder are lower in older adults (0.1%) than in the younger population (1.4%) (Robins & Regier, 1991). Late-onset bipolar disorder appears to be related to a higher risk of cerebrovascular disease (Subramaniam, Dennis, & Byrne, 2006), a fact consistent with the findings of white matter hyperintensities in individuals who develop bipolar disorder for the first time in later life (Zanetti, Cordeiro, & Busatto, 2007).

Personality

Previously focused on personality's relative stability or change throughout middle and later adulthood, late-life personality research now seeks to examine the correlates of personality with other aspects of functioning such as health-related behaviors and cognitive processes.

TRAIT THEORY

Trait theories regard personality as an entity that reflects constitutional or innate predispositions. The most widely accepted current approach, the Five Factor Model (FFM; McCrae, 2002) proposes a set of basic personality traits thought to affect the course of an individual's life (McCrae & Costa, 2003). An increasing body of evidence points to the personality-health relationship at least through the midlife years. Low conscientiousness is related to higher rates of weight gain in early adulthood (Pulkki-Raback, Elovainio, Kivimaki, Raitakari, & Keltikangas-Jarvinen, 2005); in middle adulthood high neuroticism in women is related to more weight gain (Brummett et al., 2006). Low scores on conscientiousness and high scores on neuroticism also relate to the likelihood of cigarette smoking (Terracciano & Costa, 2004). Changes in hostility in adulthood predicted a series of health-related behavior including obesity, failure to exercise, high-fat diets, social isolation, and poor health (Siegler et al., 2003).

SOCIOEMOTIONAL SELECTIVITY THEORY

In contrast to the FFM, Socioemotional Selectivity Theory (SST) proposes a dynamic interaction between emotions and personality, proposing that with increasing age, adults become more focused on maximizing the emotional rewards of relationships and less interested in seeking information or knowledge through their interactions with others. The recognition that there is less of a future ahead prompts older individuals to reduce their networks and only associate with those who are closest to them

(Carstensen, 1991). Therefore older adults prefer relationships that are emotionally fulfilling.

Socioemotional selectivity theory bears similarities to the principle of selective optimization with compensation (Baltes & Baltes, 1990). According to this theory, older adults select activities and pursuits that align with their functional abilities and personal goals. They also optimize their strengths and abilities through their chosen activities and seek to compensate for functional losses. This pattern of maximizing gains and minimizing losses represents a path toward optimizing well-being.

PSYCHOSOCIAL THEORY AND IDENTITY

A life-span orientation is provided by Erikson's psychosocial theory (1963), which focuses on the development of the self or ego through a series of eight stages. In this theory, each stage of development is defined as a crisis in which particular stage-specific issues present themselves as challenges to the individual's ego, reflecting a complex interaction of biological, psychological, and social forces characteristic of that period of life. The "crisis" is not truly a crisis but rather a critical period for either a positive or negative resolution of a particular psychosocial issue.

The characteristic theme of later adulthood is that of Ego Integrity versus Despair, a period during which the individual is preoccupied with existential issues regarding life's meaning and the ability to face death with acceptance. Erikson's theory also postulates that throughout adulthood, identity remains a central theme of development.

Expanding on Erikson's views of identity, identity process theory (Whitbourne, 2002) proposes that identity interacts with an individual's approach to the changes associated with the aging process. Changes in physical and cognitive functioning throughout middle and later adulthood stimulate the individual to incorporate age-related changes into identity. Although older adults may attempt to minimize the extent of these changes at least for a time, eventually these changes become integrated into self-concept. These changes typically occur through a sequence of phases over time, a set of "multiple thresholds" (Whitbourne & Collins, 1998). Identity appears to be related to a number of key adaptational processes. Self-esteem is higher in older adults who are able to integrate experiences into their identities in a flexible manner, a process referred to as identity balance. However, high levels of self-esteem are also found in older individuals who avoid thinking about negative changes associated with aging experiences and instead maintain their identity in a consistent manner (Sneed & Whitbourne, 2003).

There are gender differences in identity as well; women are more likely than men to focus on experiences that potentially could threaten their stable view of the self over time (Skultety & Whitbourne, 2004). Indeed, the ability to resist negative stereotypes of aging may be related to longevity. Older adults who managed to avoid adopting negative views of aging (which may be seen as a form of identity assimilation) in one study lived 7.5 years longer than those individuals who did not develop a similar resistance to accommodating society's negative views about aging into their identities (Levy, Slade, Kunkel, & Kasl, 2002).

Geropsychologists recognize that personality plays an important role in adaptation to normal age-related changes, whether viewed in terms of traits, adaptive processes, or views of the self. Interactions between personality and physical changes, cognition, health, and social context influence the individual's ability to maintain positive feelings of well-being throughout the later adult years.

Research Methods

Because aging is intimately tied up with the passage of time and cannot be manipulated as an independent variable, gerontological researchers are unable to make causal inferences about the effects of age. Similarly, the realities of aging may also pose complications for each type of study design used in research, whether longitudinal, cross-sectional, or sequential.

LONGITUDINAL STUDIES

The longitudinal design involves following people over time. Of greatest value are longitudinal studies that involve observations spanning years if not decades. Although longitudinal research has many advantages, it is limited by the problem of subject attrition over time. As the number of subjects dwindles, data analysis becomes increasingly difficult. Even if there is an adequate number in the total sample, there may be too few to permit more refined analysis of other variables such as sex, social class, race, or health.

Loss of participants also creates difficulties when the investigator wants to draw inferences from the sample to the population as a whole. The people who disappear from the sample do so for a variety of reasons such as poor health or death, lack of motivation, or an inability to continue in the study because they have moved from the area or are otherwise unreachable. Those who remain in the study may differ on all or some of these factors. Conclusions made about the survivors, therefore, may not apply to the general population.

Similar to the cohort issues that can confound analysis of cross-sectional studies (mentioned below), major historical events such as the Great Depression, the Holocaust, or the 2005 Hurricane Katrina can broadly affect the experiences of the populations under study. As a result, generalizations may be limited concerning one cohort of individuals living through one historical epoch.

CROSS-SECTIONAL STUDIES

Cross-sectional designs, in which researchers compare the performance of people who differ in age, also suffer from attrition problems. Regarding variables of interest, older individuals tested may represent a more selective group than those who are no longer alive or who decline participation. In addition, cross-sectional findings can be biased by cohort differences that can obscure or exaggerate age effects. Along these lines, awareness of the era in which a particular study was conducted is important to ensure that the results are generalizable to current older adults. For example, the results of a longitudinal study carried out in the 1990s on adults followed from ages 40 to 65 may no longer apply to current samples of 40- to 65-year-olds, who are 10 or 20 years younger than the original sample and perhaps healthier or better educated.

Consequently, cross-sectional findings must be carefully examined to ensure that they are based on samples that are comparable on key characteristics that could have a bearing on the outcomes. For example, a cross-sectional study investigating white matter volume in young, middle-aged, and older adult samples found significant age differences but failed to control for education (Brickman et al., 2006). Although the findings may nevertheless be valid, the lack of control on a variable that could be related to the main question of interest compromises conclusions about age and white matter volume.

SEQUENTIAL STUDIES

Overcoming the shortcomings of longitudinal and cross-sectional studies are sequential designs, which attempt to tease apart the effects of age from those of cohort or other possible confounds. Sequential designs literally involve a "sequence" of studies, such as a cross-sectional study carried out twice over a span of 10 years, a method known as a cross-sectional sequences design. In addition to allowing for replication of the findings derived from simpler cross-sectional or longitudinal designs, sequential designs also make it possible to draw age gradients that expand the length of a longitudinal study from, for example, 10 to 20 years when two separate cohorts are followed over a 10-year period. The consumer of gerontological research should carefully evaluate results from studies in which survivor effects or cohort differences have not been controlled or estimated.

One example of a sequential study comes from an investigation of psychosocial development in two cohorts of adults spanning the college years through ages 42 and 53, respectively (Whitbourne, Sneed, & Sayer, 2009). Although age changes were observed in the quality of "industry," defined in Eriksonian theory as a sense of identification with society's work ethic, these varied by birth cohort. Research on intelligence throughout adulthood conducted by Schaie and colleagues has also shown the importance of following multiple cohorts over multiple time periods in order to separate the effects of changes within individuals from the effects of exposure to environmental conditions associated with social and historical events (Schaie & Zanjani, 2006).

RESEARCH CHALLENGES

Research designs, no matter how cleverly engineered, are not worthwhile if there are not enough subjects to yield valid results. Recruiting older adult research participants can be a challenge: While they are less likely than younger groups to work full time, older adults can be less enthusiastic about research participation. Difficulties in arranging travel to the study site, concern over possible frustration and fatigue from study procedures, and failure to meet eligibility criteria due to co-occurring medical or psychological illnesses can all hinder recruitment in gerontological studies. Unsuccessful subject recruitment can stymie progress on even the most pressing research questions.

Finally, when researchers evaluate the quality of research evidence in gerontology, it is important to keep in mind that the instruments must be utilized with people who are likely to vary in ability, educational background, and sophistication with research instruments. Furthermore, the age of samples used to establish the validity and reliability of the measures must also be considered. Tests designed for young adults may not be appropriate for older adults and thus the standardization samples for studies in gerontology must be carefully examined. For further discussion, see Edelstein and Koven's chapter, "Older Adult Assessment Issues and Strategies," in this volume.

Conclusions

Older adults form a heterogeneous group and represent several decades of life more often marked by change than by stability. However, as discussed in this chapter, most in this group weather the vagaries of aging with resilience and often even success. Understanding the later years from the biopsychosocial perspective requires consideration of biological, psychological, and social processes. Biological processes in later adulthood involve decreased capabilities in attention, processing speed, and working memory but also the building of adaptive strategies to compensate for decrements. Psychological adaptations include growing awareness of the self as an aging individual and responding to both the losses and the comforts that come with the later years. Dealing with the transition to retirement or the death of a spouse, as well the pleasures of becoming a grandparent and enjoying even richer relationships with lifelong companions, are social processes particular to late-life.

Although complicated grief and depression are significant mental health problems in this group, subthreshold depressive symptoms are far more prevalent. Vigilance to the often atypical presentation of depressive symptoms is required for every clinician working with older adults.

The most important principle in understanding older adults, however, is to resist ageist stereotypes. Geropsychologists need to be sensitive not only to the challenges older adults confront but also to their adaptive capacity.

PART II

Skill Competencies

FOUR

Older Adult Assessment Issues and Strategies

Barry Edelstein and Lesley Koven

There are numerous age-related changes (e.g., biological, physiological, psychological, medical) that can challenge the clinician's assessment knowledge and skills. The task of assessment can be daunting if one is unprepared for these challenges, which is the case for many students and practicing clinicians who have not been trained and educated to provide services to older adults. In 2006 a model for professional geropsychology training and a set of aspirational competencies for the practice of professional geropsychology was delineated by the representatives to the National Conference on Training in Professional Geropsychology (also known as the Pikes Peak Conference). Assessment is one of the five major competency domains addressed by the conference participants. These domains are further broken down into two subdomains: knowledge base and skills.

The purpose of the present chapter is to provide some of the basic assessment-related knowledge that would be expected of a psychologist who is preparing to work with older adults, and to provide suggestions for addressing some of the challenges of assessing older adults. The chapter was prepared with the assumption that clinicians at the novice and intermediate levels would particularly benefit from the information.

Consideration of Age-Related Biological and Physiological Changes

Competent geropsychologists are able to consider the presentation of patients in light of age-related biological and physiological changes in older adults. Accommodations must be made for deficits resulting from these changes so that assessment performance and validity are maximized and not compromised. In addition, competent geropsychologists should be aware of age-related changes so that manifestations of these changes are not mistaken for symptoms of mental disorders or result in deficits that are mistakenly classified as non-normative.

SENSORY CHANGES

The visual and auditory systems undergo significant changes with aging. In addition to modifying one's assessment strategy to accommodate for changes in vision and hearing, it is necessary to consider the impact of these changes on older adults' psychosocial and cognitive functioning.

The most common age-related change in the visual system is presbyopia, or the loss of focusing ability when viewing objects at near distances. Presbyopia typically begins in the teenage years but typically is not noticeable until the 40s, when an early symptom is often difficulty reading fine print up close (Jackson & Owsley, 2003). Although loss of visual acuity is partly caused by lens opacity and changes in the optical properties of the lens, it is also likely that much vision loss is accounted for by neural deterioration along the visual pathway associated with aging (Weale, 1987). Most older adults require the use of corrective lenses, and clinicians should encourage clients to bring glasses with them to the assessment. Further, written materials and self-report instruments should be printed in a relatively large font (e.g., size 14) to facilitate accurate sight of the text. Older adults' visual acuity tends to be best with high levels of ambient light and low levels of glare (caused by exposure to scattered light or the presence of an extraneous light source, such as oncoming headlights when driving; Jackson & Owsley, 2003). Materials printed on glossy paper will cause increased glare in an assessment session and likely result in decreased visual acuity and diminished performance.

Hearing loss is perhaps the most expected and accepted age-related sensory change. However, hearing impairment can lead to profound consequences for older adults' social, functional, and psychological well-being. Of all the age-related changes in the auditory system, those that have the greatest impact on older adults' ability to hear occur in the cochlea (Howarth & Shone, 2006). There is little redundancy in the cochlea, with each region transducing a particular frequency of sound. Thus, the loss of any small collection of cells will have a noticeable effect on the older adult. Most commonly, age-related cell death in the cochlea leads to mild to moderate hearing loss that primarily affects the ability to hear mid to high frequencies bilaterally (Schuknecht & Gacek, 1993). Age-related changes to the number, size, and neurochemical makeup of cells in the auditory processing center of the brain may affect interpretation of sound and understanding of speech (Pichora-Fuller & Souza, 2003). In particular, older adults may have difficulty following conversations in environments with background noise, as more complex auditory processing is required. Older adults may also experience hearing impairment due to accumulated insults to the cochlea caused by noise or ototoxic drugs (e.g., aminoglyco-sides; Howart & Shone, 2006).

Clinicians working with older adults should inquire directly about the presence of hearing impairment and should routinely ask clients if they are adequately hearing questions and instructions during the assessment. Clues that an older adult may have hearing deficits include loud speech, repeated requests for the examiner to repeat instructions, a tendency to keenly watch the speaker's mouth, or tilting one's head in the direction of the sound. To minimize the difficulty older adults have at hearing normal speech when there is substantial background noise, a quiet environment is essential for interviewing or testing. Because older adults tend to have greater difficulty hearing high frequency sounds, female clinicians may attempt to lower the pitch of their voices. Speech should be slowed and of moderate loudness, without shouting or over-articulation, which can distort speech and make lip-reading more difficult. Older adults should be encouraged to bring hearing aids to assessment sessions; however, clini-cians should be aware that hearing aids do not overcome all hearing prob-lems and that many hearing aids can be uncomfortable for the user due to excessive amplification of loud sounds (Howart & Shone, 2006).

Age-related visual and hearing impairments can have a significant impact on older adults' quality of life and everyday functioning. Clinicians should be aware of this relationship and consider sensory changes when conceptualizing older adults' mental health or psychosocial functioning. For example, decreased visual acuity may lead older adults to give up previously enjoyed leisure activities such as reading or handicrafts, or avoid outings for fear of falling. Similarly, decrements in peripheral vision and susceptibility to glare often lead older adults to limit or stop driving, poten-tially resulting in decreased social opportunities, isolation, or feelings of dependency. Older adults' ability to successfully perform independent activities of daily living (IADLs) may also be limited by age-related visual changes. Managing medications, paying bills, shopping for groceries, and cooking are all affected by decrements in visual acuity. Hearing impair-ments may lead to a desire to avoid social gatherings or increased conflict between family members as a result of miscommunications or increased effort required to communicate.

COGNITIVE CHANGES

Aging individuals experience decline in a variety of cognitive domains. Most notably, older adults tend to have decrements in processing speed, episodic memory (memory for autobiographical details), working memory, and abstract reasoning abilities (Peters, 2006; Salthouse, 2004) relative to younger adults. Although there is great interindividual variability in the magnitude of cognitive decline and the impact of cognitive decline on real-world functioning, clinicians working with older adults should be aware of these common age-related cognitive changes and make efforts to accommodate for them during the assessment.

Extensive research has documented declines in multiple cognitive abilities associated with age. However, little consensus exists as to why these changes occur. The influential processing speed theory of aging (Salthouse, Hancock, Meinz, & Habrick, 1996) suggests that age-related declines in cognitive performance can largely be accounted for by changes in decision-making speed. Evidence to support this theory comes largely from studies demonstrating a relation between general slowing and various indices of age-related brain integrity, such as head size and white matter integrity (Greenwood, 2007). Alternatively, Hasher and Zacks (e.g., Hasher, Stolzfus, Zacks, & Rypma, 1991) have argued for an inhibition theory of cognitive aging, suggesting that declines in the ability to inhibit attention to irrelevant stimuli lead to the decrements seen across multiple cognitive domains.

Older adults often continue to perform well on the cognitive tasks of living despite declines in many underlying cognitive capabilities. That is, performance on laboratory tasks that measure cognitive functioning does not map perfectly onto performance of many important day-to-day tasks that older adults encounter (Stern & Carstensen, 2000). Specifically, "the more an everyday problem is complex, ambiguous, and dependent on a variety of skills, the weaker the relation between traditional measures of intelligence and performance" (Stern & Carstensen, 2000, p. 24). Experience-based procedural and declarative knowledge tend to be well preserved in later life (Baltes, Staudinger, & Lindenberger, 1999; Blanchard-Fields and Hess, 1996). Thus, older adults are likely able to adapt to declines in particular cognitive abilities by capitalizing on their reserves (optimization; Baltes et al., 1999), and altering the nature and pattern of their activities (compensation; Baltes et al., 1999).

Clinicians working with older adults can accommodate for age-related cognitive changes by considering the following suggestions during their assessment. Clinicians may wish to allow extra time for their interviews or assessments with older adults to accommodate their clients' slower response time to interview questions and standardized assessments. The session should be conducted in a quiet room with few extraneous stimuli that may distract older adults' attention from the tasks of the assessment. To accommodate for memory problems, clinicians may wish to provide written reminders of appointments, homework assignments, or important details of the session. If it appears that a client is having difficulty with recall of his or her personal or medical history, clinicians should gather information from additional sources (e.g., review of medical records, interview of family members, etc.).

Medical Factors to Consider When Assessing Older Adults

A competent geropsychologist appreciates the potential roles of medical factors (e.g., medications, physical disease) in the presentations of older adult clients when conducting a clinical assessment, conceptualizing the presenting problems, establishing diagnoses, formulating treatment plans, and evaluating progress.

PSYCHOLOGICAL MANIFESTATIONS AND CORRELATES OF PHYSICAL DISEASE

Medical illnesses can produce a range of psychiatric symptoms. In most cases, there are two mechanisms by which this occurs. The first and most obvious mechanism is that poor emotional adjustment to physical illness leads to the psychiatric disorders. For example, physical illness in already vulnerable individuals may result in depression and anxiety as a result of the associated challenging life events, losses, and disability. The second mechanism involves a more specific pathophysiological process whereby the psychiatric symptoms and disorders become direct sequelae of the physical illness. That is, the diseased brain directly causes psychiatric symptoms (Lyketsos, Kozauer, & Rabins, 2007). Further, physical illness can lead to difficulties with sleep, appetite, physical functioning, and the ability to socialize, which can exacerbate existing psychological symptoms and limit the effectiveness of psychological interventions.

There is a high frequency of psychiatric symptoms in almost all neurological conditions that affect the central nervous system. It is expected that over the course of a neurological illness (e.g., Parkinson's disease, multiple sclerosis, Huntington's disease, Alzheimer's disease), the vast majority of individuals will experience affective symptoms, cognitive impairment, and disturbances of perception (e.g., hallucinations, delusions) at some point (Lyketsos et al., 2007). Psychological symptoms often accompany the traditional neurological symptoms of the neurological illness (e.g., motor dysfunction, language impairment, involuntary vocalizations), yet can cause greater impairments to functioning and quality of life (Lyketsos et al., 2007). In the following section, we provide some examples of psychological symptoms associated with a variety of physical disorders.

Parkinson's disease has been associated with cognitive dysfunction, affective disorders, psychotic symptoms, impulse control problems, and problematic dysfunctional behaviors (Marsh, 2008). Depression is quite common in Parkinson's disease, with a prevalence of 40% to 50% over the course of the illness (Marsh, McDonald, Cummings, & Ravina, 2005). Most commonly, the depressive symptomatology resembles dysthymia or subsyndromal depression rather than major depression, with irritability, anxiety, anhedonia, and withdrawal from day-to-day activities being the most prevalent symptoms (Marsh, 2000). Although not well studied, anxiety and panic attacks are also common concomitants of Parkinson's disease, with potential worsening of these symptoms associated with low levels of L-dopa (Lyketsos et al., 2007).

Mood disturbances are also the most common psychological symptom in the post-stroke population, affecting 30% to 50% of patients within the first year (Dafer, Rao, Shareef, & Sharma, 2008). In addition to affecting quality of life, post-stroke depression has been associated with excess disability, cognitive impairment, poor response to rehabilitation, slow physical recovery, and increased mortality (Dafer et al., 2008). The etiology of post-stoke depression is complex and likely involves a combination of lesion location and other predisposing factors such as previous history of depression, limited coping skills, lack of social support, other cardiovascular risk factors, amount of disability, and so on. There is little consensus about the types of brain lesions that lead to post-stroke depression; however, there appears to be an association between basal ganglia and frontal lesions and incidence of depression (Carson et al., 2000).

Although estimates vary, the risk of depression in individuals with chronic obstructive pulmonary disease (COPD) appears to be approximately 2.5 times that of healthy controls (van Manen et al., 2002). Both direct (neuronal damage caused by hypoxia) and indirect (reaction to losses associated with the illness) mechanisms appear to lead to the higher rates of depression in this population (Stone & Nici, 2007). Anxiety is also common in COPD due to the hypoxia and dyspnea that accompany the disease (Frazer, Leicht, & Baker, 1996). Further, the rapid and shallow breathing often associated with anxiety and panic can lead to exacerbation of COPD symptoms.

Depression is the most common psychological manifestation of diabetes mellitus, with the prevalence of major depression estimated at 11% and sub-syndromal depression at 31% in patients with Type I and Type II diabetes (Anderson, Freedland, Clouse, & Lustman, 2001). Poor metabolic control and functional impairment due to diabetic complications (e.g., neuropathy, retinopathy, sexual dysfunction) can cause or worsen depressive symptoms and lessen response to antidepressant treatment (Lustman & Clouse, 2005). Further, the burden of caring for diabetes, including adhering to dietary restrictions and monitoring glucose levels can significantly diminish quality of life and lead to affective disturbances (Katon, 2008). In cardiovascular disease, the prevalence of depression is also quite high (estimates of 20%; Carney & Freeland, 2008) and is often the result of existential concerns, restrictive diet/exercise guidelines, and functional losses. Similarly, osteoarthritis leads to a two- to threefold increase in depression relative to individuals with no arthritis (Lin, 2008). Pain, functional losses, and restricted activity levels all contribute to the incidence of depression in individuals with arthritis.

MEDICATION USE AND PSYCHOLOGICAL SYMPTOMS

Medication use by older adults requires particular attention in the assessment process in light of the increased use of medications and the greater sensitivity of older adults to the therapeutic and adverse effects of medications. Older adults' use of prescription and over-the-counter medication is significantly higher than in any other age group. Older adults represent about 15% of the U.S. population but use one-third of all prescription drugs and 40% of all nonprescription drugs (Maiese, 2002). In a meta-analysis of polypharmacy (i.e., the use of multiple medications and/or the administration of more medications that are clinically indicated), Hajjar, Cafiero, and Hanlon (2007) found that community-based older adults took an average of two to nine prescription medications per day. Specifically, 57% of older U.S. women took more than five prescription medications and 12% took more than 10 prescription medications. Also, a study of rural community-living older adults found that over 90% took at least one and almost 50% took two to four over-the-counter medications (Stoehr, Ganguli, Seaberg, Echement, & Belle, 1997). When these data are compounded with altered pharmacokinetics, pharmacodynamics, impaired renal function, reduced hepatic blood flow and liver size, increased body fat, decreased lean body mass, changes in receptor sensitivity due to aging, and increased number of medical conditions, the chances of adverse drug reactions and interactions are greatly increased (Rolita & Freedman, 2008).

Many commonly prescribed medications and over-the-counter medications can cause psychological symptoms. For example, oral corticosteroids (e.g., prednisone) used to reduce inflammation in asthma and COPD can cause depression, mania, and psychotic symptoms (Brown, Kahn, & Nejtek, 1999). Hallucinations, illusions, insomnia, and psychotic symptoms are possible side effects of several antiparkinsonian agents (Salzman, 2005). Beta-blockers used to treat hypertension and cardiovascular disease can cause confusion, depression, delusions, paranoia, disorientation, agitation, and fatigue (Salzman, 2005). Over-the-counter cough and cold medications can cause psychological side effects. Specifically, anticholinergic antihistamines (e.g., Benadryl) can cause cognitive dysfunction and hallucinations, and medications with pseudophedrine (e.g., Sudafed) can cause insomnia, hallucinations, and agitation (Rolita & Freedman, 2008).

Unique Presentation of Mood and Anxiety Disorders in Older Adults

Competent geropsychologists are aware of the differences in depressive and anxiety symptoms of older adults relative to those of younger adults (Knight, Karel, Hinrichsen, Qualls, & Duffy, 2009). In some cases, clinicians are encouraged to look beyond the criteria of the *Diagnostic and Statistical Manual of Mental Disorders* (4th ed.; *DSM-IV*) in their assessment of depression and anxiety in older adults, as these criteria may not always be an accurate reflection of the range, magnitude, and characteristics of mental disorders in this group (e.g., Jeste, Blazer, & First, 2005). This is particularly the case when assessing older adults who are experiencing symptoms of depression or anxiety that are below the threshold required for diagnosis but are nonetheless contributing to significant impairment in functioning.

In older adults with major depression, the symptoms of moderate to severe depression are similar to those experienced by middle-aged adults if there are no comorbid conditions (Blazer, Bachar, & Hughes, 1987). However, there may be subtle differences in symptom subtypes by age. For example, melancholic depression, characterized by extreme loss of pleasure in most activities and lack of reactivity to pleasurable stimuli, appears to have a later age of onset than nonmelancholic depression, with psychomotor disturbances being more common in older adults (Parker, 2000; Parker, Roy, Hadzl-Pavlovic, Wilhelm, & Mitchell, 2001). Some investigators have attempted to identify subtypes of depression that represent the most common experience of geriatric depression. A "depression without sadness" is thought to be more common in older adults than younger adults (Blazer, 2003), as is a depletion syndrome, characterized by withdrawal, apathy, and lack of vigor (Adams, 2001). Older adults with depression report lower levels of dysphoria, fewer ideational symptoms (e.g., guilt, suicidal ideation), and higher levels of somatic complaints, anxiety, memory loss, and cognitive impairment than younger adults (Birrer & Vemuri, 2004; Fiske & Riley, 2008).

The symptoms and characteristics of anxiety disorders tend to be consistent across age ranges (Stanley & Beck, 2000). However, a number of differences have been reported in the content of older adults' worry and anxiety relative to younger adults. For example, older adults with phobias are more likely to have fears of inanimate stimuli, such as lightning or heights, whereas younger adults are more likely to be afraid of animals (Jeste et al., 2005). The content of worry and fears likely reflects developmentally appropriate themes across the life span, with older adults reporting more worry about mental decline, illness, well-being of family, and inability to care for self, and younger adults reporting more worry about finances and family (Kogan & Edelstein, 2004; Wetherell, Le Roux, & Gatz, 2003). In general, consideration of contextual factors and potential age-related differences in the experience of anxiety among older adults is important.

Jeste et al. (2005) argue for the need for age-appropriate diagnostic criteria that distinguish between anxiety disorders and behaviors that are secondary to reality-based factors. For example, he suggests that an older adult with diminished physical abilities or eyesight who is avoiding social gatherings may appear to have social anxiety disorder. However, a more thorough assessment may indicate that the individual's avoidance reflects an appropriate or adaptive fear of going out at night or into cities where he or she could be a victim of crime.

Conduct of Assessment

The competent geropsychologist can adapt his or her approach to assessment depending on the characteristics of the older adult patient and the context in which the assessment is occurring (Knight et al., 2009). One's approach to assessment is largely determined by one's assessment paradigm. An assessment paradigm has been defined by Haynes and O'Brien (2000) as "a set of principles, beliefs, values, hypotheses, and methods advocated in an assessment discipline or by its adherents" (p. 10).

One's assessment paradigm consequently determines the questions one addresses, the assessment methods and instruments employed, and the integration and use of assessment results (Edelstein, Martin, & Koven, 2003). Two relatively distinct ends of the paradigm continuum are represented by the more traditional and more intrapsychic (e.g., trait-oriented, psychodynamic) and a more environmentally based applied behavior analysis approach. The distinction between these two approaches becomes increasingly important as one works with older adults with cognitive impairment. One can distinguish between these two paradigms with regard to their philosophical assumptions about descriptions and causes of behavior. In general, traditional approaches tend to "explain" behavior on the basis of individual dispositional characteristics or traits, which are inferred from observed behavior and self-reports. Behavioral approaches, in general, "explain" behavior by describing the conditions under which the behavior occurs. More emphasis is placed on the variables that are controlling the behavior of interest, and less inference is required with the behavioral approaches because the focus is on behavior.

A second distinction between traditional and behavioral assessment paradigms corresponds to the difference between the idiographic and nomothetic approaches to assessment popularized by Allport (1937). The idiographic approach leads one to focus on the uniqueness of the individual, whereas the nomothetic approach leads one to consider the commonalities among several individuals. Using an idiographic approach, an individual's behavior is assessed through methods and instruments that are selected on the basis of the individual and the context in which the individual behaves. For example, an older adult whom nursing home staff report is exhibiting symptoms of depression might be assessed via direct observation, report by others (staff), and self-report methods. Direct observation would focus on the reported problematic behaviors (e.g., social isolation, slowed motor behavior, infrequent engagement in previously rewarding behaviors, early morning awakening, reduced frequency of eating, crying, irritability). One might administer a self-report depression assessment instrument (e.g., Geriatric Depression Scale) and focus on responses to individual items rather than the total score. Staff members may be asked to record the frequency or duration of problematic behaviors. The individual would likely be interviewed with regard to the problematic behaviors and other problem domains. One typically does not compare the assessment results with those of other individuals, although for purposes of communication with staff, one might report a total score on the depression scale, for example. However, for the most part, the criteria or standards used by the clinician are individually determined. Mischel (1968) noted that behavioral assessment involves an exploration of the unique or idiosyncratic aspects of the single case, perhaps to a greater extent than any other approach.

Nomothetic assessment typically relies upon standardized assessment instruments that often employ the self-report method. Results of assessment are compared against a large, representative, normative sample. The individual's score is then interpreted in light of how numerous other individuals scored on the same instrument.

One can also combine traditional and behavioral approaches, which is often the case. As noted in the preceding example, one could administer a test of depression, use the total score to make a judgment about whether the individual is depressed, and use the individual item responses to characterize the individual in terms of the experience and expression of depression.

Older adults with cognitive impairment offer a unique challenge to the clinician, particularly if one has relied exclusively on a nomothetic approach. The nomothetic approach becomes increasingly ineffective as the reliability and validity of self-reported information provided by the older adult diminishes with increased cognitive impairment. Consequently, the understanding of behavior must be ascertained by the overt behavior of the individual. One must shift from a more nomothetic approach that focuses on personality and cognitions to a more behavioral and contextual approach to understand behavior. The clinical question now shifts from "why is this person behaving in this fashion" to "under what conditions does this behavior occur" (Edelstein et al., 2003).

Use of Screening Instruments

In consideration of the time available for assessment, the ability of older adults to remain motivated, demands on attention, and limited willingness of some individuals to undergo psychological assessment, one must be prudent in selecting assessment methods and instruments. In addition, one must consider the incremental validity of each assessment method or instrument that is selected beyond the first that is employed (Garb, 1984; Sechrest, 1963). That is, one must consider whether supplementary assessment contributes to the description, understanding, or prediction of the behavior of interest. Screening instruments enable one to consider incremental validity by casting a broad net within circumscribed problem domains. They also permit an expedient hypothesis testing approach that minimizes the time and effort required of the clinician and older adult, as compared to the administration of lengthy, multidimensional tests (e.g., MMPI-II) or fixed batteries.

Screening instruments are available for a variety of problem domains, although the two most frequently examined are probably depression and cognitive impairment. These are frequently assessed with screening instruments because they often co-occur and because depression can impair performance on cognitive assessment instruments. In the latter case, the performance on tests of cognitive skills can reflect greater impairment than is actually the case. Screening instruments are not limited to the self-report method. Clinicians and facility staff can complete rating scales when the patient is too cognitively impaired or communication is difficult (e.g., GRID Hamilton Rating Scale for Depression, Williams et al., 2008).

A variety of cognitive screening instruments have been published, with the Mini-Mental State Examination (Folstein, Folstein, & McHugh, 1975) being the most popular. Nevertheless, it has its limitations (Roper, Bieliauskas, & Peterson, 1996; Tombaugh, & McIntyre, 1992) and has recently been copyrighted, which may diminish its popularity. Two more recent, and arguably better, instruments that were developed for the detection of mild cognitive impairment are the St. Louis University Mental Status (SLUMS) examination (Tariq et al., 2006) and the Montreal Cognitive Assessment (MoCA; Nasreddine et al., 2005). Both have preliminary support for their reliability and validity. If performance on a cognitive screening instrument is impaired, one can pursue more formal neuropsychological assessment, neuroimaging, or both. Recent reviews of cognitive screening instruments (Cullen et al., 2007) and cognitive screening methods (e.g., Woodford & George, 2007) have been published.

Several depression screening instruments have psychometric support for use with older adults, including those developed for younger adults (e.g., Beck Depression Inventory, Dura, Stukenberg, & Kiecolt-Glaser, 1990; revised Center for Epidemiological Studies – Depression Scale, Eaton, Muntaner, Smith, Tien, & Ybarra, 2004; Hospital Anxiety and Depression Scale, Bjelland, Dahl, Haug, & Neckelmann, 2002), and those developed specifically for older adults (e.g., Geriatric Depression Scale, Yesavage et al., 1983). See Edelstein et al. (2008) for a review of these and other instruments. Assessment instruments also are available for assessing depression in cognitively impaired individuals (e.g., Cornell Scale for Depression in Dementia, Alexopoulos, Abrams, Young, & Shamoian, 1988). As with cognitive screening, the results of depression screening may suggest the need for more thorough depression assessment utilizing multiple methods (e.g., self-report, report by others, direct observation) and sources of information (e.g., family members, institutional staff).

Ultimately, one must consider whether the methods and instruments employed have treatment utility if treatment is the goal of assessment. That is, do these methods and instruments contribute to a better outcome than one would have without them (cf., Hayes, Nelson, & Jarrett, 1989)?

Psychometric Considerations for Selection of Assessment Instruments

The competent geropsychologist can identify psychometrically sound assessment instruments for the evaluation of cognition, psychopathology, and personality to inform the assessment and intervention processes (Knight et al., 2009). Most adult psychological assessment instruments have been developed with younger adult populations. This is the population with which the psychometric characteristics of the instruments have been examined for norm-based instruments, and this is the population with which the norms have been established. Regardless of the population with which an instrument is developed, consideration of the important psychometric properties of instruments (e.g., validity and reliability) from which one is choosing is crucial if one expects reliable and valid assessment results. This knowledge is particularly important when working with older adults, as relatively fewer instruments have been developed for them, and because many of the instruments developed for use with younger adults have been used increasingly often with older adults. In the latter case, an appreciation for the potential consequences of such applications is important.

NORMS

Age norms are critical for the interpretation of most, if not all, norm-based assessment instruments. Age-related differences often appear on tests of psychological functioning and cognitive skills. The risk of using young adult norms for older adults is the misinterpretation of results. Indeed, in some cases the use of inappropriate norms could yield age-related biases (cf. Edelstein et al., 2003). For example, in light of the age-related cognitive changes experienced by many older adults, the use of young adult norms could lead one to conclude that an older adult's cognitive skills are relatively more impaired than one would conclude with older adult norms. Similar problems can arise with tests of psychopathology (e.g., depression) that were created for younger adults.

RELIABILITY

All forms of reliability (e.g., test-retest reliability, internal consistency) can potentially be affected by age-related population differences (e.g., cognitive functioning, life experiences, physical functioning, cohort differences). When examining the psychometric characteristics of assessment instruments for use with older adults, one should hold the instruments to the same standards as one would with younger populations. Most important, reliability estimates should be available with older adult populations.

CONTENT VALIDITY

Content validity is a judgment of the extent to which an assessment instrument adequately samples the content domain of interest (Cronbach, 1971). This may well be the most important type of validity one should consider when selecting assessment instruments for older adults. The item domain must be appropriate for the age group, as the experience and presentation of various symptoms of psychopathology can be different across groups. For example, depressed older adults are generally less likely to report dysphoria, guilt, and suicidal ideation than younger adults and more likely to report hopelessness, helplessness, and nonsuicidal thoughts of death than younger adults (Fiske & O'Riley, 2008). Older adults are also more likely to report somatic symptoms (e.g., fatigue, insomnia) than younger adults. Note that these reported somatic symptoms cannot be attributed entirely to physical disorders (Norris, Arnau, Bramson, & Meagher, 2004). As noted earlier, even the nature of self-reported fears differs between younger and older adults (Kogan & Edelstein, 2004).

CONSTRUCT VALIDITY

Construct validity is an important feature of an instrument that is developed to measure some attribute or quality of an individual that is not operationally defined (Cronbach & Meehl, 1955). Such attributes or qualities are typically conceptualized as constructs, which are used to account for variation in performance on an assessment instrument (Cronbach & Meehl, 1955). The nature of the construct and its relation to performance can change with age (e.g., intelligence; Strauss, Spreen, & Hunter, 2000). Construct validity should be established with the age group for which the assessment instrument is intended (cf. Kaszniak, 1990).

CRITERION-RELATED VALIDITY

Predictive and concurrent are the two types of criterion-related validity. As with other types of validity, these must be established with the age group being addressed. Predictive validity is an index of the extent to which an assessment instrument can predict behavior. When establishing predictive validity, the age of the individuals whose performance is being predicted must be similar to the age of the individuals in question. Concurrent validity is an index of the relation between an instrument of interest and another assessment instrument that purports to measure the same construct. As with predictive validity, when concurrent validity is being established, the criterion being used (e.g., performance on a test of the same construct) must be established with the age group in question.

Assessment of Diminished Capacity

Older adults are considered to have capacity (i.e., be competent) in all domains (e.g., consent to treatment, make financial decisions) unless adjudicated as incapacitated. With increasing age, one faces an increasing number of situations in which one's capacity can be challenged due to physical or medical problems. Over half of older adults suffer from at least one chronic disease, and many suffer from two or more. For example, in 2005–06, 52% of men and 53% women aged 65 years and older reported having hypertension, and 43% of men and 54% of women reported having arthritis (Federal Interagency Forum on Aging-Related Statistics, 2008). Chronic diseases, and even the medications taken for them, can require medical decisions for which some older adults lack capacity. Many older adults who are cognitively impaired are challenged by medical and financial decisions, voting, driving a car, or completing a last will and testament. Clinicians who work with older adults are often asked to assess older adults for capacity, often because the older adult's medical decision-making capacity has been questioned. Though clinicians have historically evaluated capacity with unstructured interviews and mental status examinations, the reliability and validity of these methods have been questioned (e.g., Marson, McInturff, Hawkins, Bartolucci, & Harrell, 1997; Rutman & Silberfeld, 1992). It is particularly important when assessing older adult capacity that the emphasis be on the functional competence of the individual (cf. Grisso, 1986, 2003; Marson et al., 2000). Cognitive assessment can be used to supplement and support information obtained through functional assessment of the skills involved in a particular capacity.

Grisso (1986, 2003) has presented a widely supported conceptual model for the assessment of capacity that is the basis for the MacArthur Competence Assessment Tool-Treatment (MacCAT-T) that was co-authored by Grisso and Appelbaum (1989). Grisso proposed a six-element model of capacity that can be used to guide one's assessment: causal, functional, contextual, interactive, judgmental, and dispositional factors. The American Psychological Association and the American Bar Association Commission on Aging recently published a first-rate guide to the assessment of older adult diminished capacity for psychologists entitled *Assessment of Older Adults With Diminished Capacity: A Handbook for Psychologists*. The authors present a very useful framework for assessing capacity and reporting the results. The framework includes the following topics: (1) Legal Standard, (2) Functional Elements, (3) Diagnosis, (4) Cognitive Underpinnings, (5) Psychiatric or Emotional Factors, (6) Values, (7) Risk Considerations, (8) Steps to Enhance Capacity, and (9) Clinical Judgment of Capacity. The book is available at www.apa.org/pi/aging/capacity_psychologist_handbook.pdf.

Testing the Limits

It is not uncommon when testing abilities to continue administering test items beyond the point that an individual has met the criterion for stopping the administration of the scale or subscale. This is termed "testing the limits." It is a method for attempting to extract as much information from the performance of an individual as possible. In some cases it is prudent to perform these tests after the entire test has been administered so as not to contaminate the standardized administration. Testing the limits can be potentially useful across a wide range of tests. For example, when requesting that an individual spell the word "world" backward when administering the MMSE, one might find that the individual is unable to do so. To test the limits one might use a different word of the same length or a word comprising fewer letters. Though the performance cannot be used in scoring the test, one can potentially reveal that the individual is capable of performing a similar task or one that is similar and less demanding. One might also test the limits when examining a person's decision-making capacity following administration of a standardized test. If the goal is to capture the individual's best performance, then testing the limits can often be quite helpful.

Referral for Additional Evaluation

The competent geropsychologist is capable of referring the older adult patient for neuropsychological, neurological, psychiatric, medical, or other evaluations as indicated (Knight et al., 2009). It is the rare clinician who has the skills and knowledge to formally assess every facet of an older adult's functioning. In some cases the presenting problems one faces can be examined at one level (e.g., screening). For example, a clinician might refer an older adult for more extensive neuropsychological or neurological examination upon determining that the individual is evidencing impairment on a cognitive screening instrument. A neuropsychologist might also refer an older adult to a neurologist for further evaluation that might include some form of imaging (e.g., MRI). The functional skills of an older person might be initially assessed with an instrument measuring activities of daily living, and then the individual could be referred to an occupational therapist for further evaluation. Finally, a geropsychologist might refer an older adult for a medical evaluation before attempting a psychological evaluation to rule out possible underlying medical or pharmacological contributions to the presenting symptoms. Most important, one must consider one's own level of expertise in assessment and seek consultation or refer patients when one's level of expertise is exceeded by the presenting problems. In most cases, a multidisciplinary approach to assessment will be the most successful.

Conclusion

The present chapter provides basic assessment-related knowledge that one would expect a psychologist who is preparing to work with older adults to have acquired. The chapter was prepared with the assumption that clinicians at the novice and intermediate levels would particularly benefit from the information. The complexity of assessing older adults should be evident from the discussion of many of the more salient factors that could potentially influence the assessment process and outcome. Clinical geropsychologists must be competent clinical psychologists, but also have a broad knowledge of age-related changes in cognitive, biological, and physiological functioning that contribute to the often unique presentation of mental disorders, and of the confounding effects of co-morbid physical disorders and medications. One must be a psychological detective who draws upon multidimensional and multi-disciplinary clues to assemble an accurate conceptualization of the presenting problem(s).

FIVE

Interpersonal Psychotherapy and Psychodynamic Psychotherapy

Gregory A. Hinrichsen

The field of geropsychology has benefited by the many contributions of researchers and practitioners who developed and refined psychotherapies for the treatment of a wide variety of mental disorders and life problems. Rich clinical formulations and innovative theories of change especially from adherents of psychodynamic psychotherapy and psychoanalysis laid the groundwork for the systematic development and testing of psychotherapies. Early on, a small body of anecdotal reports and observational studies provided suggestive evidence that older adults could benefit by psychotherapy. Some geriatric mental health professionals interwove gerontological perspectives to elucidate unique aspects of providing psychotherapeutic services to older adults (Kastenbaum, 1963; Kastenbaum, Barber, Wilson, Ryder, & Hathaway, 1981). However, not until the 1980s did results of some well-designed studies appear in the professional literature that provided evidence for the utility of a number of psychotherapies for older adults. Currently a corpus of studies indicates that many psychotherapies that were originally developed for younger populations are effective for older people (Gatz et al., 1998; Mackin & Arean, 2005; Scogin, Welsh, Hanson, Stump, & Coates, 2005). A variety of literature reviews and meta-analyses indicate that many psychotherapies are as powerful in the treatment of late-life depression and other disorders in older adults as they are in younger adults (Scogin & McElreath, 1994). A parallel literature exists on the efficacy of psychotropic treatment of late-life mental disorders (Mackin & Arean, 2005).

This chapter reviews two psychotherapeutic approaches that have been adapted or developed for use with older adults: interpersonal psychotherapy (IPT) and psychodynamic psychotherapy. The chapter discusses the elements of these psychotherapeutic interventions, needed adaptations for older adults, and evidence of their efficacy. This review is mindful of competencies outlined in the Pikes Peak Model competencies (Knight, Karel, Hinrichsen, Qualls, & Duffy, 2009), which urge geropsychologists to "apply individual, group, and family interventions to older adults using appropriate modifications to accommodate distinctive biopsychosocial functioning of older adults and distinct therapeutic relationship characteristics (p. 213)" as well as to "use available evidence-based treatments for older adults (p. 213)." An emphasis on the use of empirically supported psychotherapies is part of broader professional developments in the last 15 years to encourage use of interventions for health and mental health problems for which evidence of efficacy exists (Chambless & Ollendick, 2001).

Interpersonal Psychotherapy (IPT)

Interpersonal psychotherapy was developed by Gerald Klerman, Myrna Weissman, and their colleagues in the 1970s. IPT was premised on empirical studies demonstrating that interpersonally stressful life events increased risk for depression (and other disorders) and that depression itself created interpersonal stresses that have enduring consequences (Weissman & Paykel, 1974). The theoretical origins of IPT are rooted in the interpersonal school of psychiatry best known by the work of Harry Stack Sullivan (1953) and also the social psychiatry movement of the 1950s and 1960s which examined the social origins of mental health problems. IPT has been used in a wide variety of clinical research studies. It has been found to be useful in the treatment of acute depression, for "continuation/maintenance treatment" of depression, with other diagnostic groups (i.e., eating disorders), with specific age groups (i.e., adolescents, older adults), and with specific clinical populations (i.e., HIV-positive patients, primary care patients). (See Weissman, Markowitz, & Klerman, 2000, for a review of studies.) IPT has been adapted from its original individual format (i.e., conjoint treatment of marital disputes, groups) and brief versions have been created. Further, IPT has gained popularity among researchers outside of the United States and in other cultural contexts (Bass et al., 2006; Bolton et al., 2003; Verdeli et al., 2003). The International Society for

Interpersonal Psychotherapy is IPT's professional home (www.interper sonalpsychotherapy.org).

STRUCTURE OF INTERPERSONAL PSYCHOTHERAPY

Interpersonal psychotherapy is typically delivered in 16, 50-minute individual sessions (Weissman et al., 2000). The three phases of treatment are these:

1. initial sessions (weeks 1–3)
2. intermediate sessions (weeks 4–13)
3. termination (weeks 14–16)

Treatment focuses on one or sometimes two problem areas. IPT's four problem areas include

- Grief (complicated bereavement)
- Role disputes (conflicts with a significant other)
- Role transitions (major life changes)
- Interpersonal deficits (difficulty initiating or sustaining relationships)

During the initial sessions, depression symptoms are reviewed with the client, a diagnosis of depression (typically major depressive disorder) is made and discussed, interpersonally relevant life events that preceded or coincided with the depressive episode are discussed, problem area(s) that will be the focus of therapy are identified, treatment goals are established, and the plan for treatment is discussed. Explicit goals and strategies exist for each of the four IPT problem areas. During the intermediate sessions, the therapist helps the client to achieve treatment goals. The status of the client's depression is regularly evaluated and reviewed with the client. During the termination phase, the end of therapy is discussed along with associated feelings about end of treatment. The extent to which treatment goals have been met, the degree to which depressive symptoms have remitted, and the need for further or other treatment (including monthly "maintenance IPT") are reviewed in termination sessions. The IPT ethos is collaboration, therapeutic encouragement and hopefulness, and psychoeducation.

INTERPERSONAL PSYCHOTHERAPY AND OLDER ADULTS

Clinical and research reports indicate that IPT maps well to problems commonly seen among depressed, older adult outpatients and is well received by older IPT clients; acute clinical outcomes are similar to those found in research studies (Hinrichsen & Clougherty, 2006). Role transitions represent the problem area most commonly seen among older adults in IPT including transitions to the care role for a family member with health problems, transition to the medical patient role with the onset or exacerbation of health problems, assumption of the role of primary caretaker for a grandchild, residential relocation, and retirement. Interpersonal disputes among older IPT clients typically include difficulties with spouse and adult child. Grief treatment addresses complicated bereavement issues. For older adults these are associated commonly with the death of spouse/partner and, less commonly, child or grandchild. Interpersonal deficits have rarely been the chief problem area for older adults seen in IPT clinical practice or research.

RESEARCH ON IPT FOR OLDER ADULTS

Although many of the IPT studies of "mixed-age" adults have included some older adults, a smaller body of research specifically has examined the acute and maintenance utility of IPT with older adults (typically at least 60 years of age or older). Several studies exist of the efficacy of IPT in acute treatment of major depression and depressive symptoms in older adults. Two small pilot studies suggest that IPT may be useful for depressed older adults (Rothblum, Sholomskas, Berry, & Prusoff, 1982; Sloane, Staples, & Schneider, 1985). Another investigation was an outpatient study of a brief form of IPT with older adults initially hospitalized for medical problems and who evidenced depressive symptoms. Compared with older adults treated with "usual care," those treated with IPT exhibited significantly fewer depressive symptoms after 6 months (Mossey, Knott, Higgins, & Talerico, 1996). Recent work has found that IPT is superior to usual care for moderately to severely depressed older adults with major depression in primary care settings but not for mildly depressed older adults (van Schaik et al., 2008).

Two studies of "continuation/maintenance" treatment of major depression in older adults have been conducted. In these studies older adults were initially treated with IPT and antidepressant medication. Those who improved were randomized to monthly IPT, medication, combination, or a control condition. Notably, over three-quarters initially demonstrated significant remission of acute symptoms (Reynolds et al., 1999). In the first study, monthly IPT, medication, and the combination significantly reduced the likelihood of relapse. In a similarly designed second study, only medication reduced the likelihood of recurrence of depression and not monthly

IPT (Reynolds et al., 2006). Speculating on the divergence of findings between the two studies, the authors noted that participants in the second study were 10 years older than those in the first study and were more likely to have cognitive impairment (i.e., perhaps older, cognitively impaired patients profit less in IPT therapy than others). However, subsequent analyses of study data found that older patients treated with monthly IPT who had poorer cognition, in fact, fared better clinically than those with better cognition (Carreira et al., 2008).

Overall, there is suggestive evidence that interpersonal psychotherapy is useful in the treatment of acute major depression and depressive symptoms in older adults yet randomized, controlled clinical studies are needed. IPT alone or in combination with antidepressant medication is useful in reducing the recurrence of depression in "young" older adults but not those of advanced years although the reasons for this difference are not entirely clear. Notably, an adaption of IPT for older adults with cognitive impairment has been developed and one hopes will be tested in clinical trials (Miller, 2009).

Psychodynamic Psychotherapy

There are many schools, branches, and emphases that come under the rubric of psychodynamic psychotherapy. Important components of many psychodynamic psychotherapies include (1) attention to the diagnostic and therapeutic power of the therapist-patient relationship (e.g., "transference" and "countertransference"), (2) understanding and therapeutic interpretation of early life experiences as they influence presenting problems, and (3) the role of psychological mechanisms and internal conflicts as they bear on the genesis or maintenance of presenting problems. Psychodynamic psychotherapies span a continuum of supportive to more interpretive emphases based on presenting problems, psychological strengths/vulnerabilities of the patient, and related factors (Bond, 2006; Leichsenring & Leibing, 2007). Some psychodynamic therapies are time limited and others are long term. Components of psychodynamic and non-psychodynamic psychotherapies overlap.

Despite the long history of psychodynamic psychotherapy as a treatment modality, fewer studies undergird the efficacy of it than cognitive and behavioral psychotherapies (and their combination), which are treatments that did not substantively begin to enter clinical practice until the 1970s. Nonetheless, a corpus of studies documents that psychodynamic psychotherapy has proven efficacy in the treatment of a variety of disorders.

A recent review by the Cochrane Collaboration found that short-term psychodynamic therapy was associated with significantly greater improvement in symptoms and social functioning than that in controls; and that improvements were maintained (Abbass, Hancock, Henderson, & Kisely, 2006).

Psychotherapy with older adults received scant attention until the last 25 years. However, a small cadre of geriatric psychiatrists (Goldfarb, 1955) integrated psychodynamic concepts into the formulation and treatment of problems of older adults, and professional groups such as the Boston Society for Gerontologic Psychiatry and its journal, the *Journal of Geriatric Psychiatry*, were a forum for the psychodynamic view of late-life problems. Others were noted for their contributions to the psychodynamics of late life (e.g., Griffin & Grunes, 1990; Gutmann, 1992; Lazarus, 1980; Myers, 1984). More recent works have provided thoughtful conceptualizations and commentary of psychodynamically relevant issues and later life (Duffy, 2004; Newton & Jacobowitz, 1999; Nordhus, Nielsen, & Kvale, 1998).

The best-known and existing studies of the efficacy of psychodynamic psychotherapy in the treatment of depression were conducted by Dolores Gallagher-Thompson, Larry Thompson, and their colleagues. They compared brief psychodynamic, cognitive, and behavioral therapies. Psychodynamic treatment was based on work by Horowitz and Kaltreider (1979) and Mann (1973). Among older adults with major depression, they found that all active treatments were associated with significant improvement compared with a waiting list control (Thompson, Gallagher, & Breckenridge, 1987). A 2-year follow-up documented sustained gains among the three treatment groups (Gallagher-Thompson, Hanley-Peterson, & Thompson, 1990). In another study they compared brief psychodynamic psychotherapy with cognitive behavioral therapy in the treatment of depressive disorders in family caregivers of infirm older adults. Both approaches proved efficacious, yet psychodynamic therapy was most useful for caregivers in the earlier months of providing care whereas cognitive-behavioral therapy was most useful for those who had been caregivers for longer periods of time (Gallagher-Thompson & Steffen, 1994). Earlier work by Steuer and colleagues (Steuer et al., 1984) found that depressive symptoms were significantly improved among older adults receiving longer-term psychodynamic psychotherapy and cognitive behavioral therapy although improvement was significantly greater for those receiving cognitive behavioral therapy. Scogin and colleagues (Scogin et al., 2005) list psychodynamic psychotherapy among six identified evidence-based treatments for depression in older adults.

Practice Implications

Both of these psychotherapeutic approaches can address individual and relationship issues that emerge typically in the context of late-life stressors, most notably health problems. A modal clinical case for geropsychologists is a depressed and anxious older woman providing care to an ailing husband and who herself is dealing with health problems. All approaches are informed by an effort to help the client better contend with current problems with the goal of improved emotional well-being including reduction of mental health–related symptoms. The client's past history including interpersonal and problem-solving strengths and difficulties inform how the therapist works with the client's current problems. A good working relationship between therapist and client is important to therapeutic progress regardless of whether therapist-client relationship dynamics are used to promote therapeutic change.

The Pikes Peak Model competences (Knight et al., 2009) urge that those who provide services to older adults develop knowledge and skills competencies in the treatment of older adults and their families. Fortunately, most psychotherapies developed for use with younger adults appear useful for older adults. Practice with older adults is also informed by knowledge of older adults and the problems usually evident in clinical practice with them (American Psychological Association, 2004).

However, much work remains to be done to better tailor existing psychotherapeutic interventions to the needs of racial and ethnic minority older adults, those with cognitive impairments, and individuals with highly complex medical and mental health needs (Karel & Hinrichsen, 2000). The Pikes Peak Model competencies therefore urge practitioners to "develop psychotherapeutic interventions based on empirical literature, theory, and clinical judgment when insufficient efficacy research is available on older adults" (Knight et al., 2009, p. 213). Efforts are required to bring psychotherapeutic services to older adults where they reside and congregate as well as to enhance residential environments, particularly long-term care facilities. A solid body of research demonstrates the powerful impact of the environment on older adults' well-being, particularly for those with reduced emotional, behavioral, and/or cognitive capacities (Lawton & Nahemow, 1973). Therefore, the Pikes Peak Model competencies urge practitioners to "demonstrate ability to intervene in settings where older adults and their family members are often seen (e.g., health services, housing, community programs) with a range of strategies including those targeted at the individual, family, environment, and system" (Knight et al., 2009, pp. 213–214).

Acquisition of skills competencies may be more challenging for practitioners who work with older adults particularly those who have not received formal training in clinical geropsychology (Qualls, Segal, Norman, Niederehe, & Gallagher-Thompson, 2002). Possession of several psychotherapy skills sets may be especially useful in best matching psychotherapeutic approach to client and problem type, regardless of the client's age. Non-geropsychology trained practitioners who possess skills in the delivery of several psychotherapies and who begin to see older adults in clinical practice can enhance competency by becoming familiar with how those therapies may be best adapted to older adults. Geropsychologists who are skilled at only one psychotherapeutic approach can potentially enhance their clinical effectiveness by acquiring another psychotherapy skill set. For example, a psychodynamically trained clinical geropsychologist could benefit by acquiring competency in the delivery of a cognitively-behaviorally informed caregiver intervention. Or, a cognitive-behavioral clinical geropsychologist could benefit by learning how to conduct interpersonal psychotherapy.

Supervision by experienced "specialists" and/or self-assessment are ways to acquire competency in evidence-based practice for older adults. In a formal psychotherapy supervisory relationship, competencies are typically assessed on an ongoing basis during supervision with feedback provided to the supervisee. In clinical research studies psychotherapeutic competency is often conducted with the use of formal rating scales to document treatment adherence (Hill, O'Grady, & Elkin, 1992). Often, however, post-licensure clinicians will make self-assessment of skills they possess in the implementation of psychotherapeutic approaches and related clinical skills. One project through the newly formed Council of Professional Geropsychology Training Programs (CoPGTP; www.usc.edu/programs/cpgtp) is development and testing of a rating instrument based on the competencies elucidated in the Pikes Peak Model. This instrument could be used for assessment of therapeutic competencies in self or other (i.e., trainee).

Conclusions

These two psychotherapeutic approaches are among several that have been found or are likely to be useful in the treatment of later-life mental health problems. Interpersonal and psychodynamic psychotherapies were developed originally for younger adult populations and later adapted for use with older adults. These therapies are consonant with the Pikes Peak

Model competencies' emphasis on the use of evidence-based treatments for older adults and interventions that address late-life caregiving issues. The challenge for those who deliver services to older adults is finding the vehicles by which they may gain training/experience to add one or more of these approaches to their clinical repertoire or acquire competence in the adaptation of psychotherapeutic approaches they possess to older adults. Acquisition of competencies to meet the health and mental health needs of an aging population is a challenge for health professionals (Institute of Medicine, 2008) for which geropsychology has much to offer.

SIX

Applying the Pikes Peak Model of Treatment Competency to the Use of Cognitive-Behavioral Therapies with Older Adults

Forrest Scogin and Andrew Presnell

It is increasingly evident that an identifiable corpus of knowledge and skills is available and required for the competent treatment of older adults. A well-supported class of treatment is the cognitive-behavioral therapies. This chapter's purpose is to examine specifically the application of Beck's cognitive-behavioral therapy (CBT) and problem-solving therapy (PST), an adaptation of cognitive-behavioral techniques, with the older adult population. The Pikes Peak Model (Knight, Karel, Hinrichsen, Qualls, & Duffy, 2009) will be used to identify the focal areas needed for competent delivery of these treatments with older adults.

The Pikes Peak Model outlines six areas to be considered in the competent application of treatment:

1. Applying interventions with appropriate modifications

2. Using evidence-based treatments

3. Developing appropriate treatments when there is a lack of evidence available

4. Proficiently employing common late-life intervention

5. Using interventions to enhance the health of diverse elderly persons

6. Intervening across settings

The sections that follow target these six areas. First, the justification for CBT and PST as evidence-based treatments for older adults is presented. Next, methods for modifying treatment as well as intervening across settings are presented together. Third, common issues that require late-life psychological interventions and the evidence-base for their application are offered. Fourth, health enhancing interventions are presented, and finally, case examples demonstrate how both CBT and PST can be used proficiently as interventions with older adults.

Evidence-Based Treatments

BECK'S COGNITIVE-BEHAVIORAL THERAPY (CBT)

Arguably the most prototypical CBT approach, though not the only one in use, was developed by Aaron T. Beck (Beck, Rush, Shaw, & Emery, 1979). The CBT premise is that many disorders and problematic issues stem from negative attitudes, cognitions, and behaviors. Through identifying these dysfunctional and maladaptive thoughts and behaviors, a client in therapy can then work to change them. The development and maintenance of these new behaviors diminishes the symptoms of the expressed disorder (Beck et al., 1979).

The application of CBT does not follow a set pattern but instead comprises a variety of techniques to elicit changes in cognitions and behavior (Beck et al., 1979). CBT begins with an introduction to the cognitive mediation theory. The client works with the therapist to collect data to either support or negate the reality of the cognitions that produce the problem. The highly collaborative nature of the therapy allows the client to build the skills necessary to cope with similar problems in the future. In addition to the cognitive tasks in CBT, behavioral and psychoeducational components enrich the therapy, providing the client with skills to improve coping and overall health. All tasks can and generally are augmented with the use of homework, allowing therapy to continue beyond the clinical site and office.

CBT has been established as an evidenced-based treatment for depression and anxiety disorders (Dobson, Backs-Dermott, & Dozois, 2000). Research is continuing to build strong cases for the use of CBT in other disorders, such as substance abuse, sleep problems, obsessive-compulsive disorder, bipolar disorder, somatization disorder, schizophrenia, and post-traumatic stress disorder. The wide variety of issues that appear to be amenable to treatment with CBT makes it a valuable modality.

Of more recent focus, CBT has been shown to be effective across a wide sample of problem areas with geriatric populations. Laidlaw and Thompson (2008) summarize the use of CBT with older adults thus: "Cognitive behavior therapy is particularly appropriate as an intervention for older adults because it is skill-enhancing, present-oriented, problem-focused, straight-forward to use, and effective" (p. 102). CBT is also flexible and allows the therapist to tailor treatment to various strengths and weaknesses present in older adults (Zeiss & Steffen, 1996). Research supporting the use of CBT with older adults is solid but not extensive. A special issue of *Psychology and Aging* (Scogin, 2007) reviews evidence-based treatments for a variety of problems commonly experienced by older adults and CBT is promi-nently featured. Additional details are provided later in the chapter.

PROBLEM-SOLVING THERAPY

There are several therapies that are a form of CBT and are unique enough to warrant separate discussion. These therapies include multimodal therapy, cognitive bibliotherapy, and problem-solving therapy. Problem-solving therapy (PST) has been the subject of some important research and is becoming increasingly popular in general, and specifically in work with older adults.

PST is a structured treatment that promotes problem solving as an active coping strategy. It uses both problem-focused and emotion-focused coping techniques to examine problems (Nezu, 2004). The problems can be dealt with in one of three ways: adaptive and rational problem solving, impulsive problem solving, and avoidant problem solving. Through breaking down the problem-solving process, individuals are able to deal with the cognitive and emotional aspects of problems. It was first proposed by D'Zurilla and Goldfried (1971) and was further developed by D'Zurilla and Nezu (Nezu, 2004). For older adults, PST provides clear steps for solving problems. Therapists help clients through four key steps:

1. Clearly defining and formulating a particular problem that is exacerbating their depressive disorder

2. Formulating a thorough list of possible solutions to the problem (usually alternatives to current coping methods)

3. Examining potential consequences of each solution and determining one to make use of based on those consequences

4. Evaluating the outcomes of the chosen solution after it has been implemented to determine whether or not to build the strategy into a routine (Moss & Scogin, 2008)

Problem-solving therapy is praised for being a pragmatic, concrete, and easy to understand treatment. As such, it is generally accepted as being easily taught to and implemented by paraprofessionals (e.g., case managers, nurses) in a broad range of settings. Numerous studies have demonstrated its effectiveness in treating many disorders in a variety of settings (Nezu, 2004). The primary evidence that directly supports the use of PST with older adults has been in the treatment of depression. Several studies have demonstrated this effectiveness (Alexopoulos, Raue, & Areán, 2003; Areán et al., 1993; Hussain & Lawrence, 1981). Ongoing research is extending the range of PST applications with older adults.

Appropriately Modifying Treatment and Intervening Across Settings

Several issues may affect psychological treatment of elders. Knight and Lee (2008) have described a useful model for work with older adults that emphasizes both potential strengths and specific challenges older clients may bring to treatment. The Contextual Adult Lifespan Theory of Adapting Psychotherapy (CALTAP) model combines an understanding of age-related decline with attention to the effects of cohort and culture. Cognitive and physical changes in older adults may present challenges that require accommodation of the therapeutic process.

As discussed in Edelstein and Koven's chapter, "Older Adult Assessment Issues and Strategies," in this volume, therapists may want to use memory aids to address working memory impairments in older adult clients, such as repeating information and allowing the client to keep notes or providing notes or audiotapes for review by the client (Knight & Lee, 2008; Zeiss & Steffen, 1996). Both CBT and PST tend to be information rich and didactic in nature and thus memory aids may be needed for some clients. Memory aids for treatment can be printed handouts or a treatment journal. For example, the session agenda can be written on a white board or a sheet of paper. For working with deficits in processing speed, the therapist will want to slow down the presentation of material, both through using small amounts of information at any one time and by allowing time for the client to absorb what is said (Knight & Lee, 2008). Another cognitive aging manifestation that may be seen in older adults is increased distractibility. Decreases in attentional capacity make it more difficult for older adults to maintain a topical progression. Active listening and careful redirection can counteract distractibility (Zeiss & Steffen, 1996). By monitoring the course of the therapeutic interaction the therapist can detect whether the client is straying from the therapeutic task. If so, at this point the therapist must use thoughtful and respectful redirection to return the process to the desired focus (Knight & Lee, 2008; Zeiss & Steffen, 1996). This can be difficult and requires a skillful bedside manner.

Sometimes cognitive impairment may severely hinder the ability of clients to follow the cognitive aspects of CBT. In these cases, a therapist might rely more on behavioral activation (BA). BA focuses on the behavioral aspects of CBT, engaging the client in pleasurable events to activate more positive emotions (Martell, Addis, & Jacobson, 2001). The primary goal of behavioral activation is to increase these positive activities and in turn increase positive reinforcement for the individual.

These cognitive issues may be particularly salient for CBT and PST. Cognitive-behavioral therapy in particular requires monitoring and recall of cognitive phenomena such as unhelpful thoughts, and this may prove challenging for some older adults. Therapists need to be mindful of their clients' capabilities and adjust accordingly.

Physical impairments are also present in many older adults. Some therapeutic activities may require adjustment for deficits in vision, hearing, and movement, such as reading or listening to psychoeducational information or participating in certain relaxation techniques that require movement. Printed materials may need to be enlarged for those with sight issues or the volume and rate of speech may need to be augmented for older adults with difficulty hearing. Sometimes, the adjustment in therapy may not be as subtle. Treatment goals, such as a return to autonomy, may be unrealistic with certain impairments (Knight & Lee, 2008). In these cases, such as after a stroke, a return to full autonomy may be medically contraindicated. Consideration of such factors is important when setting goals for therapy.

There are other considerations for implementing therapy appropriately with older adults. First, it is necessary to understand the client's culture. Culture can affect the understanding of aging itself, the help-seeking behavior of the individual, and the meaning of the therapeutic relationship. By carefully listening to the client and obtaining information about the client's cultural background, the therapist can tailor interventions to the client's needs. An excellent description of the role culture can play in the therapeutic relationship with older adults is presented in the CALTAP model of Knight and Lee (2008). Please also see Tazeau's chapter, "Individual and Cultural Diversity Considerations in Geropsychology" in this volume.

Second, when treating older adults, consideration of the setting in which therapy will take place is necessary. Older adults may receive treatment in primary care clinics or other medically necessitated settings such as nursing homes or rehabilitation centers (Brenes, Wagener, & Stanley, 2008). One consideration in these settings is that sessions will often need to be brief. Consequently, Brenes et al. (2008) suggests using written materials and telephone contacts to supplement the therapy. Another important consideration when working in a medical setting is communication with the other professionals working with the client. The coordinated interdisciplinary care of the older adult is optimal and arguably should be the standard of care. Please also see Emery's chapter, "Integrative Care Models", in this volume.

Working with older adults can be challenging due to the many factors that play a role in treatment implementation. Conversely, older adults bring strengths to the process such as wisdom and maturity that can make such work immensely rewarding. For more in-depth and specific information on treatment considerations and adjustments, refer to Knight and Lee (2008), Zeiss and Steffen (1996), and Moss and Scogin (2008).

Common Late-Life Interventions

DEPRESSION

Depression is a common mental health issue for older adults. A CBT manual specific to the treatment of late-life depression has been created by Laidlaw and colleagues (Laidlaw, Thompson, Dick-Siskin, & Gallagher-Thompson, 2003). It provides a very comprehensive set of instructions for therapists. The manual divides the treatment into three parts. In each part, there is an outline of the tasks that the client and the therapist are to be working toward. For example, it suggests that early sessions focus on educating the client on the therapeutic process; middle sessions focus on changing negative, automatic thoughts; and late sessions focus on preparing for termination and relapse prevention (Laidlaw et al., 2003).

Cognitive-behavioral therapy is the most researched therapy in the treatment of geriatric depression. Eight out of the nine studies examined by Scogin et al. (2005) supported traditional CBT as a beneficial treatment for older adults with a depressive disorder or clinically significant depressive symptoms.

Problem-solving therapy has also been established as an evidence-based treatment for older adults with depression. Slightly modified versions of PST (as part of more comprehensive treatment services) have received a great deal of attention recently for proving successful in reducing depressive symptoms in primary care (Bruce et al., 2004; Lin, Katon, & Von Korff, 2003). Scogin et al. (2005) found three studies that established support for the use of PST with depressed older adults. Two of these studies employed the commonly used protocol by Nezu, Nezu, and Peri (1989).

LATE-LIFE ANXIETY

Anxiety is a prevalent psychological issue in older adults and is associated with a host of negative health outcomes (Ayers, Sorrell, Thorp, & Wetherell, 2007).

Of the various anxiety disorders, generalized anxiety disorder (GAD) is the most clearly researched in treatment literatures. The general protocol of CBT in the treatment of GAD involves psychoeducation, awareness training, relaxation techniques, cognitive restructuring, and exposure therapy (Brenes et al., 2008). Wetherell and colleagues (2005) have developed a CBT protocol for use specifically with older adults. This protocol focuses less on purely cognitive tasks, making it more accessible to many individuals, and instead focuses on skills training. The skills are taught as modules that can be chosen to match the idiosyncratic symptom expression of the individual. Modules include problem-solving skills, cognitive restructuring, and progressive muscle relaxation, to name a few (Wetherell, Sorrell, Thorp, & Patterson, 2005). An advantage of this approach is that modules can be selected as a way to tailor the treatment, by using those that focus not only on specific symptoms but also on strengths and weaknesses of the client (Beck, 2008). For more details on this model, refer to the protocol (Wetherell et al., 2005).

Cognitive-behavioral therapy has been supported in the literature as a treatment for late-life anxiety. Ayers et al. (2007) found nine studies that met criteria for an evidence-based review that supported treatment with CBT. The review also found evidence for the use of relaxation training alone, which is a behavioral component of CBT. Four studies in the review supported the use of this treatment. Ayers et al. (2007) caution that the research on late-life anxiety is still not extensive, though results to date have been solid and suggest that further research is necessary.

INSOMNIA

The likelihood of developing chronic insomnia increases 25% to 50% after the age of 65 (Lichstein & Morin, 2000). Fortunately, several interventions have proven efficacious for older adults with insomnia. CBT has a strong evidence base in the treatment of insomnia in older adults (McCurry, Logsdon, Teri, & Vitiello, 2007). The intervention strategy that uses tenets of CBT is known as multicomponent CBT treatment. Cognitive-behavioral interventions are used to challenge thoughts and beliefs that contribute to poor sleep in older adults (Cook, Nau, & Lichstein, 2005). Often the negative thoughts lead to anxiety that makes it hard to sleep. Relaxation techniques are taught to counteract the anxiety felt at the time of sleep for persons experiencing insomnia (Lichstein, 2000). The intervention also focuses on sleep hygiene, structured relaxation techniques, and sleep scheduling (Morin & Espie, 2003). Sleep hygiene is the identification of both problematic behaviors and stimuli as well as sleep-enhancing stimuli

(Cook et al., 2005). For example, the therapist may help a client realize that watching television while waiting to fall asleep may actually be an impediment to sleep. Finally, sleep scheduling can be accomplished either through sleep restriction (Friedman et al., 2000) or sleep compression (Lichstein, Reidel, Wilson, Lester, & Aguillard, 2001). For example, sleep restriction limits the time spent in bed without sleep in an effort both to reset normal sleep cycles and to keep sleep time scheduled. Though the techniques differ slightly, they both aim to restructure the behaviors that lead to sleep disruption. For a more comprehensive overview of the use of CBT for insomnia in older adults, see Morin and Espie (2003).

The treatment of insomnia as described above, which combines cognitive and behavioral techniques, has yielded effective results (Morin, Colecchi, Stone, Sood, & Brink, 1999). Indeed, the results of an evidenced-based review of insomnia treatments in older adults found seven studies that established the multicomponent CBT as an evidenced-based treatment (McCurry et al., 2007). The review found no studies that did not support the effectiveness of this treatment. The mean effect size for the treatment of insomnia in older adults with CBT was found to be .97 relative to the control groups. Research has also independently supported the various components of the insomnia treatment described above. Individually, sleep scheduling techniques have found the greatest empirical support in older populations (Lichstein et al., 2001; McCurry et al., 2007).

PSYCHOTIC SYMPTOMS

The utility of CBT in the treatment of schizophrenia-related symptoms has been established in the literature. However, use with older adults has yet to receive much attention. One group has developed a manual for the use of CBT with older adults experiencing psychotic symptoms (Granholm et al., 2005). This treatment, called Cognitive Behavioral Social Skills Training (CBSST), incorporated modifications targeted for the challenges of working with older adults. The treatment focuses on using CBT to challenge thoughts and social skills training to manage symptoms (McQuaid et al., 2000). This therapy is tailored to older adults through using memory aids and focusing on content relevant to the age group, such as role-playing talking to the doctor. Results from this study suggest that the use of CBSST improved skill acquisition and cognitive insight in the participants relative to the treatment-as-usual control (Granholm et al., 2007).

Health Enhancing Interventions

CAREGIVER DISTRESS

A common issue that must be dealt with in an aging population is that of caregiver distress. Caring for individuals with Alzheimer's or other severely debilitating disorders can be difficult. The treatment of caregivers focuses on alleviating depression, anxiety, negative emotionality, and excessive burden (Steffen, Gant, & Gallagher-Thompson, 2008). Though most therapeutic interventions for caregivers are based on cognitive and behavioral therapies, they are often labeled as skill-training or stress-management classes to better appeal to the population (Burgio, Hardin, Sinnott, Janosky, & Hohman, 1995). However it is presented, components of CBT are generally included to address the anxiety and depression that often arise in caregivers (Gallagher-Thompson & Coon, 2007).

In a review of the available studies on caregiver interventions, Gallagher-Thompson and Coon (2007) distinguished between treatments that may have shared some elements of CBT and the use of strict CBT. The review calculated the effect size for the strict CBT studies to be a robust 1.20, the highest of the grouped treatment modalities they reviewed. This review established CBT as an evidenced-based treatment for caregivers that results in lower depression and anxiety scores in caregivers (Gallagher-Thompson & Coon, 2007).

Bourgeois et al. (2002) and Gallagher-Thompson et al. (2000) conducted studies using the PST treatment developed by D'Zurilla (1986). Bourgeois et al. (2002) found that caregiving spouses who received PST showed more improved mood and lower strain than the control groups at the end of treatment and at follow-up. Gallagher-Thompson et al. (2000) found that PST led to increases in cognitive and behavioral coping when compared to a wait-list control. Though these studies do not establish PST as an evidence-based treatment for caregiver distress, they point to a verdant future area of research.

GRIEF

Grief and bereavement may be experienced more often by older adults, but this does not make the experience any easier. CBT can be used to treat problematic grief, also known as complicated grief, in older adults. Gallagher-Thompson et al. (2008) state that use of the Dual Process Model (Stroebe & Schut, 1999) is appropriate within a CBT framework. The Dual Process Model suggests that adaptive coping with grief occurs through loss-oriented coping and restoration-oriented coping. CBT may play a role in facilitating "oscillation," or the shifting back and forth between the two coping methods. Shear et al. (2001) developed a manualized treatment for complicated grief that incorporates CBT techniques—namely, exposure, homework assignments, and mindfulness techniques—with interpersonal psychotherapy. Matthews and Marwit (2004) have suggested the use of more straightforward CBT treatment. They believe dysfunctional thoughts and behaviors that are maintaining the grief can be challenged and new coping strategies can give the client the tools to achieve the positive goals set in therapy.

There is little research supporting the strict use of CBT in the treatment of complicated grief in older adults. The work of Shear and colleagues (2001, 2005) has included older adults and the results have supported the use of the manualized treatment. Though not empirically based, Gallagher-Thompson et al. (2008) and Matthews and Marwit (2004) both draw on considerable experience in making recommendations that the use of CBT appears promising and appropriate in the treatment of complicated grief.

PAIN MANAGEMENT

The use of CBT can often lead to reduction in reports of pain in older adults. A model for treatment of older adults with chronic pain that is relatively new in the literature is geriatric multimodal cognitive-behavioral therapy (GMCBT; Cipher, Clifford, & Roper, 2007). This model is flexible in taking into account the abilities and preferences of the client, incorporating any number of techniques such as psychopharmacology or occupational therapy (Clifford, Cipher, Roper, Snow, & Molinari, 2008). GMCBT focuses early on establishing themes for motivating the client, such as being a leader or hardworking, and uses these to cognitively anchor assessments of problematic behaviors. As an example, someone who has been a leader in his or her past can be motivated by using an appeal to lead by example in dealing with the current situation. For a standardized manual for the implementation of GMCBT, see Cipher, Clifford, and Roper (2007).

The use of CBT for pain management in older adults is sparsely researched. The results to date have been positive, with findings indicating diminished reports of pain (Cipher et al., 2007; Cook, 1998; Reid, Otis, Barry, & Kerns, 2003). Drawing on the expansive literature supporting the effectiveness of CBT in treating chronic pain in the general population (Morley, Eccleston, &Williams, 1999) as well as the results of the aforementioned studies, the use of CBT for pain management in elders appears promising.

POSITIVE AGING

Positive aging is an emerging area of study with older adults. It refers to an approach to aging that includes promoting positive attitudes, engaging in healthful behavior, and engaging fully in one's life. Hill and Mansour (2008) discussed the use of CBT in promoting positive aging. CBT can be used both to challenge the negative thoughts, behaviors, and attitudes that can detract from positive aging as well as to instill new positive habits and thoughts. By addressing the dysfunctional thoughts and fears associated with aging and instilling new and positive habits, CBT can be used to lead to more successful and enjoyable aging. For example, CBT can be used to develop a focus on "positives" in one's life. Through reframing a person's perspective to a more optimistic outlook, a practitioner can help the client approach the changes and challenges of aging in a more adaptive manner. To review a more comprehensive presentation of the use of CBT techniques for the development of positive aging habits, see Hill and Mansour (2008).

Applying Interventions

The chapter has provided an overview of cognitive-behavioral therapy and problem-solving therapy as well as some considerations for adjusting these therapies to meet the special needs of older adults and the evidence base for their use in the treatment of specific disorders and issues. This information provides the building blocks of competency. However, it is the application of this knowledge to meet the idiosyncratic needs of an older adult that demonstrates competency. Following are two case studies that demonstrate CBT and PST treatment with an older adult.

COGNITIVE-BEHAVIORAL THERAPY: A CASE EXAMPLE

Mr. James was a 77-year-old African American male seen at a small rural primary health care clinic. Mr. James was referred to the clinical psychology graduate student psychotherapist by the nurse practitioner who was providing his medical care. The nurse practitioner had diagnosed him as depressed and had begun an antidepressant; she also wanted him to be treated via psychological means, specifically CBT. The nurse practitioner and psychotherapist maintained close collaboration throughout the course of Mr. James's treatment.

Mr. James was a widower who lived alone in his home of many years with the support of two adult daughters who lived in the same county.

Mr. James had little formal education and evidenced limited literacy but was smart in the ways of the world, affable, and quick of wit. He had spent most of his life as a farm laborer and logger, and the physical demands and danger of his work had left him scarred and worn. He had multiple medical comorbidities including diabetes, coronary heart disease, and arthritis. His left foot had been amputated due to diabetic complications. He received home health care and consistent with this approach his psychotherapy was also delivered in-home and occasionally over the telephone.

Mr. James reported to his therapist that he had been feeling down for the past couple of years as it had become increasingly difficult for him to get about and take care of himself. He described himself as pretty useless. Nonetheless, he maintained his deep spiritual and religious beliefs, indicating that his life was "in God's hands" and that whatever he was going through was part of a larger plan. His limited mobility and finances made attendance at church services difficult and this was a source of considerable frustration for him.

During the initial visit Mr. James was orally presented the 15-item Geriatric Depression Scale (GDS) to determine the severity of his depression symptoms. He scored 9, indicative of moderate depression. Further discussion with him revealed the oftentimes difficult differentiation of depression symptoms from medical conditions seen in older adults with multiple chronic medical conditions. For example, fatigability, sleep problems, and loss of interest in activities were recursively caused by his medical conditions and the depressive episode he was experiencing. He denied any suicidal thoughts and asserted that this would be against his religious beliefs. Mr. James also was administered the MMSE as a brief cognitive screen and received a score of 23. The lower score was attributed partly to his lower literacy and it was felt by the therapist to underestimate his abilities.

Formal CBT was begun during this initial 1-hour session following the manual developed by Laidlaw, Thompson, Dick-Siskin, and Gallagher-Thompson (2003). The CBT model was presented to Mr. James using a drawing on a piece of paper showing the reciprocal relations between behavior, thought, physiology, and emotion. He seemed to fully grasp that the work with his psychotherapist would target the cognitive and behavior aspects. Following the presentation of two examples of the connection of thoughts, behavior, and emotion, the session was concluded with the agreement that it would take about 16 to 20 meetings to get through the CBT "course."

Following the dictum to "slow down the process to speed up the progress" two sessions were devoted to orientation to treatment and ample time was set aside for "visiting" to provide opportunities for a strong alliance to form. Beginning with session three, the idea of unhelpful thoughts was introduced. Mr. James seemed to have some trouble in engaging in the meta-cognitive tasks of monitoring and evaluating his thoughts and thus it was determined to move quickly to behavioral activation strategies and return to more purely cognitive techniques in later sessions. Mr. James readily agreed to the premise that engaging in more meaningful and pleasurable activities would help him feel better and start an "upward spiral." However, both he and his therapist knew the challenges that his physical, financial, and social support limitations would place on the identification of such activities. Mr. James's therapist was aware of his fervent religious beliefs and had gained access to free copies of the "Bible on Tape." She suggested that one daily pleasant event could be a set-aside period of listening to these tapes. He readily engaged in this activity and seemed pleased that his therapist had not rejected his belief system. During other early and middle sessions, several additional meaningful activities were collaboratively identified and the means by which to engage in them were problem solved. These included talking on the phone or receiving visits from his grand-and great-grandchildren and watching birds at a bird feeder. The therapist was able to help Mr. James link activation with feeling better through repeated inquiry about how he felt during and after such activities.

Periodic administration of the GDS showed that Mr. James was experiencing a decrease in depression severity from 9 to 7 to 4 over the course of treatment. Mr. James's daughters, who occasionally participated in CBT sessions with him, also noticed an improvement in his affect as did his nurse practitioner. During the final phase of treatment the therapist revisited unhelpful thoughts and thought-monitoring activities, but Mr. James continued to have difficulty in engaging these techniques. Rather than belabor the issue, the therapist continued with behavioral activation as the core technical aspect of the treatment. A deep and meaningful alliance developed between Mr. James and his therapist that presented some challenges at the time of termination. The fact that there had been a predetermined stopping point established early in treatment made this a bit easier on both parties. Two follow-up sessions were scheduled at 1 and 3 months following the end of treatment. At these sessions the therapist reviewed behavioral activation techniques with Mr. James and assessed his depression. It was gratifying to see that he maintained his gains and continued to evidence relatively low depression scores.

PROBLEM-SOLVING THERAPY: A CASE EXAMPLE

Mrs. Collins was a 70-year-old White female self-referred to the university-affiliated psychological clinic. Mrs. Collins had read an article in the local newspaper about research and services being conducted at the clinic for caregivers. Mrs. Collins was the primary caregiver for her moderately demented husband. She indicated that she was experiencing considerable stress related to her caregiving role. She described feeling a mixture of sadness, guilt, anger, and entrapment. Indeed, it was very difficult for Mrs. Collins to arrange for the initial session due to concerns about leaving her husband at home even for short periods of time unless someone was there to oversee his activities.

During the initial session, the therapist learned that Mrs. Collins had suffered a significant stroke 5 years earlier that limited her mobility and strength but did not significantly impair her cognition (her MMSE was 29). She had also had a knee replacement and experienced significant osteoarthritis. Assessment of her depression suggested that she met criteria for minor depression.

The therapist determined that a problem-solving approach would be useful for Mrs. Collins given the caregiving challenges she faced. Moreover, problem-solving therapy (PST) has proved useful in controlled trials with caregiving samples (Schulz et al., 2003). The therapist used the PST manual developed by Nezu, Nezu, and Perri (1989) to guide her intervention activities. Accordingly, during the initial sessions an orientation to the treatment was offered and examples of how the PST approach had been used with caregivers were presented to Mrs. Collins. She indicated that this approach was exactly what she was looking for and expressed an eagerness to tackle some of her disconcerting problems.

Mrs. Collins and her therapist collaboratively decided on an important but potentially solvable problem as their first target: Creating time for Mrs. Collins to be away from home to take care of things including personally satisfying activities such as having her hair done, attending church services, and of course, coming to problem-solving sessions. In discussing this issue, the therapist learned that Mrs. Collins was reasonably convinced that her husband would have catastrophic reactions if she spent "too much" time away from him and that others would not know how to adequately care for him because they did not know his quirks and routines. Nonetheless, therapist and client engaged in the seven-step process that represents the core of PST (Arean & Huh, 2006). This took place over the course of several sessions.

1. Problem orientation or how one views his or her ability to cope with a problem

2. Identification of the problem in a concrete and specific fashion

3. Goal definition with achievable outcomes

4. Brainstorming or the generation of alternative solutions without judgment of potential effectiveness

5. Decision making or choosing a course of action based on cost-benefit analyses

6. Solution implementation

7. Solution verification or evaluating the success of the action

For Mrs. Collins, the goal was to be able to make her traditionally scheduled (for over 20 years) salon appointment 75% of the time. She was currently attending about 25% of the time. Mrs. Collins generated about 10 alternative solutions although it was difficult for her to refrain from pointing out the shortcomings in each. Mrs. Collins decided that among the alternatives, that of asking her next-door neighbor of over 30 years if he would sit with her husband for the 2-hour span each Friday was the most likely solution. The implementation involved role-playing her approach to this beloved neighbor and overcoming her reluctance to be a burden on him and risk a cherished friendship, all understandable and legitimate concerns. Mrs. Collins decided to take the risk and approach him and was surprised to learn that her neighbor had actually been thinking about ways he might be able to help his friends but had not approached them because he didn't want to intrude. Starting the next week, Mr. Collins enjoyed his friend's company each Friday as they had a long history of friendship. Tracking of this particular problem (several others were also addressed during the course of intervention) revealed that she was able to attend her appointments at the targeted level.

Conclusions

We conclude this chapter by offering some suggestion on routes by which to achieve competence in the delivery of cognitive-behavioral therapy and problem-solving therapy with older adults. In addition to a solid grounding in adult development and aging, we recommend careful reading of major treatment protocols, specifically Laidlaw et al.'s *Cognitive Behavior Therapy With Older People* (2003) and Nezu et al.'s *Problem-Solving Therapy for Depression* (1989) and Hegel and Arean's (2003) *Problem-Solving Treatment for Primary Care: A Treatment Manual for Depression*. Another aid in developing general competency is study of video demonstrations of psychotherapy with older adults. For example, we are aware of four relevant videos developed by the American Psychological Association, featuring Bob Knight demonstrating adjusting psychotherapy for working with older adults, Peter Lichtenberg demonstrating his multimodal approach to the treatment of late-life depression, Sara Qualls demonstrating the treatment of Alzheimer's disease through caregiver family therapy, and Gregory Hinrichsen demonstrating interpersonal psychotherapy for older adults with depression. These individuals are leaders in the training of geropsychologists and these videos provide examples of competent practice with older adults. These videos do not demonstrate CBT or PST specifically but demonstrate the issues encountered in work with older adults. They also provide excellent models for the important therapeutic tasks of alliance development, providing support, and establishing treatment goals. Another means for gathering information in pursuit of competence is attendance at continuing education (CE) offerings focusing on geropsychology practice. Exemplars in this regard include the University of Colorado at Colorado Springs 2-day intensive conferences on geropsychology topics. Focal topics have included depression, decision-making capacity, and aging families and caregiving. The American Psychological Association and its Committee on Aging recently presented a 1-day CE workshop entitled "What Psychologists Should Know About Working With Older Adults" as part of the annual convention. All of these sources contained information on the application of CBT and PST with older adults. These sources are particularly useful for those at the post-licensure level. Supervision of clinical work by a specialty trained geropsychologist is probably the premier opportunity for competence but we realize this is most realistic for predoctoral, internship, and postdoctoral levels of training. Moreover, very few of these specialty programs exist, especially at the predoctoral level.

How do you know when you have achieved competence in the delivery of psychological services to older adults? This topic is covered more extensively in other chapters of this book, but we can offer a couple of suggestions from our experiences in conducting clinical research. The gold standard for assessing skill and competence in CBT delivery is the Cognitive Therapy Scale (CTS; Young & Beck, 1980). This scale contains 17 items and is rated by listening to audiotapes or viewing videos of psychotherapy sessions. Two subscales of the CTS are General Therapeutic Factors and Specific Cognitive Techniques. Example items from the former are "Agenda" and "Interpersonal effectiveness"; examples from the latter are "Focusing on key cognitions or behaviors" and "Homework." We have used this scale in our CBT investigations and have found it a useful supervisory and teaching tool. For the person interested in developing CBT competence, the CTS could be used as self-rated tool to determine strengths and areas of needed improvement. For PST, a comparable tool is the Problem-Solving Treatment for Primary Care Adherence and Competence Scale (PST-PAC; Hegel, Dietrich, Seville, & Jordan, 2004). This scale contains seven items, six of which correspond to the problem-solving stages. The seventh item rates the overall therapist performance, taking into account problem complexity and the client.

One of the most important components of competence in any skilled endeavor, including the use of CBT and PST with older adults, is staying current with developments in the field. One of the major premises of the evidence-based practice movement is that if practitioners do not stay up-to-date with empirical knowledge, their clinical performance will deteriorate over the years after their training (Sackett, Richardson, Rosenberg, & Haynes, 1996). The growth of work in aging and mental health is dramatic and it can be a challenge to digest even a portion of what is available. As scientist-practitioners and committed professionals, we owe our clients competent delivery of psychological services, and this is not an easy task. We hope this chapter helps current and future providers reach this goal.

SEVEN

Integrative Care Models

Erin E. Emery

One in four older adults has a significant mental disorder (Jeste et al., 1999). These disorders, including depression, anxiety, and substance abuse, frequently co-occur with physical illnesses, either as precipitating or exacerbating factors, and are associated with increased risk of multiple physical health problems and mortality in older adults (Karel, Ogland-Hand, & Gatz, 2002). In fact, depression is evident in 39% to 47% of older adults being treated for cancer, heart attack, or stroke and has been associated with increased mortality from multiple diseases (Ariyo et al., 2000). Not surprisingly, this interaction of mental and physical illness is associated with increased rates of health care resource utilization (Callahan, Hui, Nienaber, Musick, & Tierney, 1994; Saravay, 1996).

Navigating the system for older adults with chronic disease and their families can be frustrating and disempowering (U.S. Department of Health and Human Services, 2001). Not only is our current system of health care difficult to maneuver through but the quality of care has been poor for older adults with diabetes, cancer, pneumonia, cardiovascular illness, urinary incontinence, falls, end-of-life care (Wenger et al., 2003), and particularly for mental health (Bartels, 2003). When each of these disorders is treated separately by providers in isolation, care for comorbid illnesses suffers even more. Furthermore, access to care is disparately limited by socioeconomic status, ethnicity, culture, immigration status, physical ability, and health insurance (Abramson, Trejo, & Lai, 2002; Banks, Buki, Gallardo, & Yee, 2007; Gauthier & Serber, 2005).

One of the reasons for this poor level of care is that there are few specialty trained health professionals to meet the needs of older adults.

In 2004, there were fewer than 7,000 board certified geriatricians (AGS & ADGAP, 2004), which is 50% of the current need, and only 19% of the anticipated need by 2030 (Alliance for Aging Research, 2002). Similarly, the number of mental health providers with specialty training in treating older adults falls staggeringly short of the need. Currently, we have only 55% of needed psychiatrists, 18% of needed social workers, and 10% of needed psychologists (Halpain et al., 1999; Jeste et al., 1999). Emery and colleagues (2007) found that only 11% of graduate training programs in the United States offer geropsychology specialty training, and few students take advantage of these programs. Even fewer programs provide training in evidence-based psychotherapy for older adults. Approximately one-third of master's level social work programs offer coursework in gerontology (Halpain et al., 1999), but only an estimated 3% of current graduate students in social work enter geriatric social work (Partners in Care Foundation, 2008). By 2030, it is estimated that we will have only 27% of the needed psychiatrists, 9% of the social workers, and 5% of the psychologists. For more on training needs, see Vacha-Haase's chapter, "Teaching, Supervision, and the Business of Geropsychology", in this volume.

Need for Integrated Care

The President's New Freedom Commission recommended that addressing the many facets of chronic illnesses might best be accomplished by increasing integrated care in primary care settings (Bartels, 2003), as it has been shown to significantly improve outcomes (Hedrick et al., 2003; Katon et al., 2002; Unützer et al., 2002). Despite the enormous boon resulting from passage of parity legislation for Medicare mental health services, reimbursement has been inadequate to support integrated care, even in the face of evidence for lower health care costs in integrated care systems (Katzelnick, Kobak, Greist, Jefferson, & Henk, 1997; Katzelnick et al., 2000). Thus, many care systems have not offered these services (American Geriatrics Society, 2005). Certainly the need for integrated care is not limited to only primary care; any setting in which older adults are receiving health care could be improved by maximizing the integration of health care providers, patients, family members, and other community members and agencies. For example, the Joint Committee on Interprofessional Relations between the American Speech-Language-Hearing Association and Division 40 (Clinical Neuropsychology) of the American Psychological Association (APA) issued a joint statement on the Structure and Function of an Interdisciplinary Team for Persons with Acquired Brain Injury (2008). The committee calls for increased integration among professionals, patients, and families in caring for those in rehabilitation settings, a majority of whom are older adults.

The American Psychological Association's Presidential Task Force on Integrated Health Care for an Aging Population (IHCAP) echoed this call in 2008, highlighting not only the health care disparities for older adults but also the lack of sensitivity to diversity in later life, lack of awareness of the roles of others in the community in late life health care, lack of trained professionals to work with older adults, and lack of communication among providers who do work with older adults. The IHCAP document outlines a model for integrated, interdisciplinary care that includes eight basic principles:

1. Integrated teams are sensitive to ageism and its influence on treatment decisions.

2. Psychologists become familiar with core roles of other health care team members.

3. Models of health care processes and beliefs may differ among team members.

4. Conflict among team members is natural and can lead to a strengthening or weakening of the team.

5. Psychologists benefit from applying conflict resolution skills to team conflicts.

6. Health care teams communicate in increasingly diverse ways.

7. Health care teams are sensitive to issues of multicultural diversity and marginalization.

8. Assessment of treatment and treatment outcomes should be ongoing.

Psychology Competencies Related to Integrated Care

Consistent with IHCAP, the importance of team functioning and integrated care are noted throughout the Pikes Peak Model competencies for geropsychologists, including knowledge of models and methods of interdisciplinary collaboration and understanding the varied components, roles, and contexts of interdisciplinary treatment of late-life mental disorders. Competent geropsychologists also have the ability to (a) address complex biopsychosocial issues among many older adults by collaborating with other disciplines in multi- and interdisciplinary teams, (b) participate in interprofessional teams that serve older adults, (c) communicate psychological conceptualizations to medical and other professionals in a concise and useful manner, (d) implement strategies for systems analysis and change in organizations and facilities that serve older adults, (e) design and participate in different models of aging services delivery (e.g., integration), and (f) collaborate and coordinate with other agencies and professionals that serve older adults.

These competencies were further broken down for the purposes of developing a measurement tool with which psychologists can assess geropsychology competence (Karel, Emery, & Molinari, in press). The following specific abilities are included in this measure: (a) understanding the theory and science of geriatric team building; (b) valuing the role that other providers play in the assessment and treatment of older clients; (c) demonstrating awareness, appreciation, and respect for team experiences, values, and discipline-specific conceptual models; and (d) understanding the importance of teamwork in geriatric settings in addressing the varied biopsychosocial needs of older adults.

Interprofessional Health Care Teams

There are many ways in which professionals from multiple disciplines work together in varying degrees of integration. Teams that work in parallel or sequential process with hierarchical leadership are considered *multidisciplinary* (Heinemann & Zeiss, 2002). Consider, for example, an acute rehabilitation team of physical, occupational, and speech therapists, social worker, psychologist, nurse, and physician. Each discipline develops their own goals for the patient and communicates them to the team in meetings; patient and family goals may or may not be incorporated into the discussion. Each discipline treats the patient separately according to its own focus of care. When disagreement arises about goals or plan of care, there may be discussion, but the physician's decision is final.

In contrast, *interdisciplinary* teams are those that work collaboratively and interdependently as equal stakeholders to achieve task-oriented and process goals of the patient, team, and organization (Heinemann & Zeiss, 2002). Goals are established jointly, and progress is evaluated as a system rather than by individual disciplines. Interdisciplinary teams incorporate shared leadership and power across all members of the team. While no single leader is hierarchically above other members of the team, there is often a "coordinator" or "facilitator" to manage the team administratively. Consider, for example, the same rehabilitation team described above,

FIGURE 7.1 **Comparing team structures.**

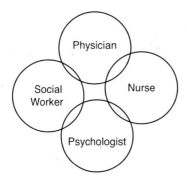

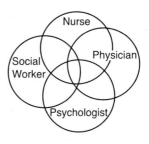

Multidisciplinary Teams work in parallel or sequential process with hierarchical leadership. Role overlap reflects each discipline's training and treatment focus rather than collaboration.

Interdisciplinary Teams work collaboratively and interdependently as equal stakeholders to achieve task-oriented and process goals of the patient, team and organization (Heinemann & Zeiss, 2002). Role overlap is designed for integrative purposes in working toward shared goals.

in which each discipline is fully aware of the others' scope of practice. A complete set of shared goals is developed incorporating the patient's plans and resources following discharge along with each discipline's evaluation of the patient's functional ability. While the nurse facilitates team meetings, each discipline's voice is equally heard and valued in decision making. Team members communicate respectfully and work toward the shared goals established by the team rather than those that serve the individual discipline or provider.

Team Development

Tuckman (1965; Tuckman & Jensen, 1977) identified four common stages in group development research from more than 70 studies; this model remains the most prominent conceptualization more than 30 years later. The four stages are forming, norming, storming, and performing.

FORMING

New teams must determine who the members will be, which patients they will serve, resources available for team and patient use, and many other content-focused decisions. Farrell and colleagues (2001) use the term *anomie* for this stage that lacks clarity and consensus, in which many team members may feel as though the development of the team is largely externally imposed by outside authority. To move toward being a performing team (low anomie), a shared culture must be developed and internalized by the members of the team, along with clearly defined roles and division of labor.

> For example, a team comprised of a physician, nurse, social worker, psychologist, nutritionist, and pharmacist may decide to focus team efforts on older adults with diabetes and depression. Questions arise about whether these patients should receive more frequent care than other patients, where and when team meetings should be held, and whether participation via conference call is acceptable for team members who are not co-located. Although the decision is made that all team members have an equal voice, the nurse, who is accustomed to deferring to the physician, has difficulty trusting that differing opinions will be acknowledged and valued. The pharmacist feels peripheral to the team and is unsure of her role. The physician's enthusiasm about the team is infectious but overwhelming for some team members.

STORMING

Team conflict is inevitable. Interpersonal style, expectations for team member participation and procedures for communicating disagreement, ideas about the process for treatment planning and implementation, along with more basic issues of start and end time for meetings must be resolved collaboratively or the team may revert to previous parallel functioning and/or disband. Psychologists' observance of team members' styles, knowledge, and application of conflict resolution skills can be highly valuable to this process.

> The Diabetes and Depression Team may agree to complete an interdisciplinary assessment but disagree about the format for that assessment. Multiple members have difficulty shifting from the previous hierarchical structure to horizontal leadership. Team members disagree about steps in the intervention process when a patient can not afford to engage with all disciplines immediately. The team psychologist reflects the interpersonal process to team members and facilitates brainstorming among team members about resolving the conflicts.

NORMING

If the team withstands the storm, normative expectations for group behavior are developed. Some norms will be explicit and specific (e.g., the team meets in the conference room on Wednesdays promptly at 8:00 A.M.), while others will be broader (e.g., when there is disagreement about a treatment plan, all team members' opinions will be welcomed equally and respectfully). These norms are to be periodically evaluated for clarity and effectiveness. As members act within the established effective norms, group cohesiveness grows. If norms are not effective, groups may become stagnant or conflicted and frustrations will arise.

> The social worker is identified as the team meeting facilitator and assures that perspectives of all team members are solicited about each patient. Team meetings are scheduled for exactly 30 minutes weekly, and conflict arises when meetings run over time. Team members collaborate to maximize efficiency. During the first meeting of each quarter, team members take the opportunity to review norms and team process, adjusting rules of engagement as needed.

PERFORMING

With experience and effective communication, as well as continuous assessment and refinement, teams will become highly skilled at collaborative decision making and treatment of patients. Group cohesiveness and morale will be maintained at a high level, and the team's functioning will appear effortlessly smooth. Each individual discipline works both individually and collectively, completing its own assessment and sharing information with all members. Teams synthesize the information with a biopsychosocial perspective that incorporates cultural, environmental, and familial issues. The synthesizing process is the most challenging and most important component of effective teams. All team members must communicate results of their assessments in a clear and concise manner in language accessible to all disciplines. Discussion must be respectful and incorporate all team members' perspectives, particularly when divergent information is presented. A comprehensive picture of the patient's needs is adopted by all members of the team and serves as the basis for the development of team goals and a plan for intervention. This may include adding members to the team to provide additional services. All team members monitor the patient's response to treatment, and bring their observations back to the team to discuss any needed modifications to the treatment plan. This process continues throughout the patient's treatment.

Mrs. Greene, a 78-year-old African American woman who is a retired executive secretary, has resided in a long-term care facility for 3 years. She moved into the facility when her uncontrolled diabetes left her with poor vision and crippling neuropathy. Despite her physical limitations, Mrs. Greene had been very active in the facility, organizing events for her fellow residents and participating in the resident council. During a diabetes team meeting, the social worker noted that Mrs. Greene had not been attending council meetings in recent weeks and had been spending much of her time in her room. The nurse observed that Mrs. Greene had been having increasingly frequent episodes of incontinence and required assistance with self-cleaning. The physician indicated that there were no infections or other medical causes for her incontinence. She also reported that Mrs. Greene's neuropathy had worsened, and she was not engaging in as much physical activity. Upon evaluation, the psychologist discovered that Mrs. Greene had always prided herself on her appearance, and was horrified at the idea of having an episode of incontinence in the presence of others. She isolated herself in her room, which led to symptoms of minor depression including decreasing attention to nutrition. The team recognized the possibility that her incontinence may be treated by strengthening her pelvic muscles, including the use of biofeedback, and consulted physical therapy. While the physical therapist worked on improving pelvic floor strength, the psychologist provided brief cognitive behavioral psychotherapy to address depressive symptoms, coping with incontinence, and maintaining adequate nutritional intake. With Mrs. Greene's consent, the social worker encouraged other residents to visit Mrs. Greene in her room to minimize isolation. The physician and nurse worked together on pain management, incontinence, and monitoring blood glucose related to her nutritional status. Disagreements arose regarding pain management, as increased medications began to impair Mrs. Greene's cognition. The team decided that it would be most effective for the psychologist to provide behavioral pain management and monitor her cognitive status as medications were titrated.

Role of the Psychologist in Integrated Care

A core competency for psychologists on teams is the ability to effectively communicate complex conceptualizations to other disciplines clearly and concisely (Knight et al., 2009). In the example of Mrs. Greene, above, the psychologist incorporated Mrs. Greene's strong self-image as someone who is "put together" being threatened by her neuropathy and incontinence, along with her pattern of declining emotionally and cognitively without social involvement, to help the team understand the reasons for Mrs. Greene's depressive symptoms. The psychologist educated the team about the serious potential effects of minor depression on individuals with chronic illness in a long-term care setting to increase engagement in the collaborative treatment of her symptoms.

The competent geropsychologist also has an understanding of common medical disorders in late life as well as of the interaction of medical illness and mental illness. The psychologist can then educate the team about psychological aspects of illness and provide evidence-based intervention for a variety of medical issues. In the case of Mrs. Greene, the psychologist was aware of psychological aspects of incontinence, diabetes, and chronic pain, which she educated the team about, and worked with the team to treat.

An additional key role for psychologists is to bring to the team knowledge of developmental processes and the diversity in aging, including normal aging versus disease process and the interaction of illness, medications, behavior, immediate environment, health care system, community, and the larger society. This knowledge can help the psychologist and the team increase their awareness of ageism that fosters the assumption that later life is characterized by disability and thus should not be treated (APA, 2004; Knight et al., 2009). Cultural expertise can also make the psychologist indispensable to the team by notifying the team of issues impacting the patient and treatment process. The psychologist on the diabetes team alerted the team to Mrs. Greene's sensitivity about being a minority in the facility and her concerns about judgment by others, particularly related to her incontinence.

The competent geropsychologist is aware of the roles of other team members, having a sense of both the educational background and the perspective of other disciplines. This includes having an awareness of the culture and history of other disciplines and ways that they have typically interacted with one another. For example, some disciplines have significant overlap in treatment focus and as such may experience some "sibling rivalry" as they address the patient's functional needs. Being aware of these relationships can help the psychologist and the team resolve conflicts when they occur. The psychologist must also provide education to the team about psychology and the perspective of the individual psychologist. This awareness of perspective extends to the patient, family, and community as members of the team. As team members come to understand each other, the psychologist may help to develop a "role map" for the team (Zeiss & Steffen, 1996) and facilitate discussion among members.

According to Janis's Group Think theory, teams risk "premature concurrence-seeking" due to fears of disrupting what is perceived to be group cohesion (Heinemann et al., 1994). The goal of avoiding conflict may come from the patient or any other member of the team. Psychologists with expertise in systems analysis and group dynamics can play an integral role in evaluating not only the patient/family/community system but also attend to the environment of care created by the team and processes within the team.

An additional role of the psychologist in integrated health care teams is to be particularly aware of issues of confidentiality. Patients and/or family members may share information with the psychologist that may or may not be appropriate to share with the rest of the team. Judgment about the level of disclosure is paramount. Further, the psychologist can heighten the awareness of the team about confidentiality related to sharing information with families and others outside the team. See Karel's chapter, "Ethics," in this volume for a more thorough discussion of confidentiality.

Patients as Members of the Team

The Institute of Medicine (IOM, 2001) reported that most patients are not involved enough in their own care to adequately manage their illness. Teams often contribute to this by meeting to discuss assessment, goals, and progress of the patient without the patient present, or without having even consulted the patient about his or her goals (Playford et al., 2000). Those with the very best interests of the patient at heart can fall into paternalistic decision making, which can compromise the therapeutic relationship (Horvath & Bedi, 2002; Newton & Jacobowitz, 1999) and increase dependency (Baltes, 1996) which is inconsistent with most team goals. The current standard for high-quality care, particularly for patients with chronic illness, is patient-centered care. Wagner and colleagues (2005) suggest that this can be achieved by assuring that patients are involved in multiple steps of the health care system, from participation in their own health care team to quality assurance and improvement initiatives. Many models have been highly effective in empowering patients to collaborate with health care professionals in the management of their own illnesses, including self-management (Gibson et al., 2003; Norris, Engelgau, & Narayan, 2001; Riemsma, Kirwan, Taal, & Rasker, 2003) and recovery (SAMHSA, 2005) models.

There are multiple issues to be aware of when involving patients in team discussions about health care. The first is language used by health care professionals; while most health care professionals have advanced degrees, 40% of older adults read at the most basic level of literacy (Kirsch et al., 1993). Although this is shifting with the aging of the baby boomer generation, 83% of the current cohort of older adults has not attended college and has a lower level of language proficiency than younger adults, which is multiplied for older immigrants (Ramírez & de la Cruz, 2003; Wan, Sengupta, Velkoff, & DeBarros, 2005). Competent geropsychologists will educate team members about the educational and language level of the patient, and assure that patients understand the content of the discussion such that they can participate effectively.

Beyond basic literacy, 50% of older adults have great difficulty understanding health care options (Hibbard et al., 1998). This too is exacerbated by lower levels of education and problems in language proficiency (Gazmararian et al., 1999). Without a shared understanding of disease causation, severity, controllability, and effectiveness of treatments, developing common goals and adhering to a treatment plan will be very challenging (Hardeman et al., 2002). Thus, when goal setting, the team must allow for discussion of patient and family perspectives and provide education about disease processes. The psychologist assures that the patient has clarity about options presented and has been encouraged to generate his or her own goals.

As we strive to include patients in their own care, we also must be aware of cultural issues that may determine the extent to which patients or their families are involved. For example, in some Asian families, it is considered most appropriate to involve the family as a surrogate for the patient in medical decision making and treatment planning, though it also is considered appropriate to obtain patient consent for this arrangement (Back & Huak, 2005). To whatever extent the patient is involved, the competent geropsychologist attends to caregivers' needs as well, particularly given that many caregivers are older adults. Caregivers are at increased risk of stress, poorer health, and increased use of health care resources (Schulz et al., 2003; Son et al., 2007). Ethnic minority caregivers with cultural obligations to manage the patient's care may be at particular risk for guilt if older family members require more assistance than they can provide. Even with these risks, psychologists recognize that caregivers, empowered with more information than ever before given the advent of the Internet, can be very strong and helpful members of the team.

Efficacy of Interdisciplinary Teams

The body of empirical evidence supporting the efficacy of interdisciplinary teams in treating older adults with multiple chronic conditions has been growing exponentially in recent years (Bruce et al., 2004; Callahan et al., 2006; Ciechanowski et al., 2004; Skultety & Zeiss, 2006). Diverse positive outcomes have been reported from studies across settings and populations of older adults. Integrated care has been linked with increased access to mental health care (Bartels et al., 2004; Hedrick et al., 2003; Liu et al., 2003), decreased length of stay in acute hospitals (Friedman & Berger, 2004), decreased pain (Weinberg et al., 2007), improved physical functioning following stroke (Strasser et al., 2008), improved treatment adherence (Katon et al., 2002; Roy-Byrne et al., 2001), increased patient satisfaction (Friedman & Berger, 2004; Weinberg et al., 2007), decreased mortality (Birbeck et al., 2006), and decreased health care expenditures (Gade et al., 2008; Katzelnick et al., 1997; Katzelnick et al., 2000; Liu et al., 2003; Sommers et al., 2000). Despite all of this evidence, particularly the latter, Medicare and other third-party payers have yet to financially support integrated care (National Council for Community Behavioral Healthcare, 2006).

Minimizing excess disability (functional impairment that exceeds expectations for the severity of the illness) has also been a key outcome of integrated teams (U.S. Department of Health and Human Services, 1999). For example, Sommers and colleagues (2000) studied 543 chronically ill older adult primary care patients to determine the efficacy of the primary care physician alone versus a team including the primary care physician, nurse, and social worker. Among other outcomes, integrated care was associated with increased social activity among older adults. It is notable that in this same study, integrated care was also associated with improved job satisfaction for service providers.

Setting-Specific Teams

Common settings for psychologists to be a part of treatment teams include primary care, acute rehabilitation, and long-term care, among many others. Models for team operation are highly varied and yield diverse outcomes. Following are examples of each, along with issues for geropsychologists to consider.

PRIMARY CARE

Most older adults seek treatment first from their primary care physician (Klapp et al., 2003; Zeiss & Gallagher-Thompson, 2003), contributing to the estimated 50% to 75% of all primary care visits focusing on a mental health concern. Most older adults also prefer to receive mental health services in primary care or religious settings (Areán et al., 2002; Chen et al., 2006;

Dupree et al., 2005). Unfortunately, physicians rarely have the training or time to adequately assess and treat mental health problems independently (Simon et al., 1999). Many mental health problems in older adults go undetected by primary care providers (Bartels, 2003), and primary care clinics rarely employ mental health providers to address this issue (US DHHS, 1999). Recognizing this need, the Surgeon General issued a report in 1999 that identified primary care as a pivotal point of care for older adult mental health. More than 10 years later, we still struggle to provide adequate mental health care in this setting.

When mental health services are provided in the primary care setting, up to 90% of patients receive the needed care, as compared to 25% receiving care when outside referrals are provided (Speer & Schneider, 2003). Further, providing mental health services in the primary care setting allows for increased integration of care, which yields better health outcomes for patients (Skultety & Zeiss, 2006) and may contribute to destigmatizing mental health treatment (Zeiss & Karlin, 2008).

A quickly growing number of interdisciplinary team programs including psychologists have been developed in recent years to address the mental health of older adults through primary care clinics and home-based care, each with a different approach to the team construction and treatment. Among them are PRISM-E (Primary care Research In Substance abuse and Mental health for the Elderly), IMPACT (Improving Mood: Promoting Access to Collaborative Treatment), Healthy IDEAS (Identifying Depression, Empowering Activities for Seniors), PROSPECT (Prevention of Suicide in Primary Care Elderly: Collaborative Trial), and most recently BRIGHTEN (Bridging the Resources of an Interdisciplinary Gero-mental Health Team via Electronic Networking).

The PRISM-E program (Primary care Research In Substance abuse and Mental health for the Elderly) employs a model in which mental health and primary care services are co-located, all mental health services are provided by licensed providers (social workers, psychologists, psychiatric nurses, psychiatrists, and master's-level counselors), and communication is documented between primary care and mental health providers about the evaluation and treatment plan for depression. Among 1,531 older adult primary care patients, integrated care was associated with a greater reduction in depression severity for those with Major Depression (Krahn et al., 2006).

Developed at the University of Washington, IMPACT (Improving Mood: Promoting Access to Collaborative Treatment) brings together the patient, a Depression Care Manager (nurse, social worker or psychologist) and primary care physician who consult with a psychiatrist to treat depression in older adults (Unützer et al., 2002). The primary components of treatment are problem-solving therapy (PST), behavioral activation, and pleasant events scheduling, along with support for antidepressant medication treatment. Participants in IMPACT have access to the Depression Care Manager for 12 months, typically including six sessions of PST. In a multisite randomized controlled trial of IMPACT, 45% of participants reported a 50% or greater reduction in depressive symptoms (Unützer et al., 2002), decreased arthritis pain (Lin et al., 2003), increase in weekly exercise (Williams et al., 2004), and improved physical functioning (Callahan et al., 2005) across ethnic groups (Areán et al., 2005) and regardless of the presence of multiple medical illnesses (Harpole et al., 2005), relative to usual care. Gains were maintained at 6- and 12-month follow-up (Callahan et al., 2005; Hunkeler et al., 2006).

Healthy IDEAS (Identifying Depression, Empowering Activities for Seniors) provides education about depression, referral to health and mental health care providers, and behavioral activation treatment for 3 to 6 months in a combination of in-home visits and telephone contacts by a case manager. The collaborative components of Healthy IDEAS extend beyond the treatment team into the community by creating relationships between community outreach workers and mental health professionals. Healthy IDEAS outcomes have included decreased symptoms of depression and pain, increased self-management/self-efficacy (ability to recognize depressive symptoms and make appropriate appointments for treatment), and less excess disability (Quijano et al., 2007).

PROSPECT (Prevention of Suicide in Primary Care Elderly: Collaborative Trial; Bruce et al., 2004) aims to prevent suicide among older adults in primary care by treating depression and reducing suicidal ideation. The intervention is designed to increase recognition of depression and suicidal ideation by the primary care physician, who then collaborates with a depression care manager (nurse, social worker, or psychologist) to provide antidepressant medication and/or brief interpersonal psychotherapy. Outcomes of this intervention include decreased suicidal ideation and decreases in major depression (Bruce et al., 2004), decreased mortality for those with diabetes (Bogner et al., 2007), and for those receiving the intervention, higher and faster depression remission rates compared with those receiving usual care (Alexopolous et al., 2005).

In each of these projects, teams operated collaboratively in a single setting. While this may be ideal, not all health care settings have this luxury. Unlike other models, the health care providers on the BRIGHTEN

(Bridging the Resources of an Interdisciplinary Gero-mental Health Team via Electronic Networking) team are not required to be co-located, or even employed by the same organization. This potential obstacle is surmounted through the novel use of a "virtual team." In this model, team members (occupational therapists, physical therapists, dieticians, nurses, psychologists, psychiatrists, social workers, pharmacists, and chaplains) are connected via electronic media including e-mail, text messaging, telephone, and/or video conferencing. Initial outcomes suggest that the program has increased identification of older adults with depression and anxiety, and increased referrals for interdisciplinary mental health treatment (Golden & Emery, 2007).

LONG-TERM CARE

Perhaps even more than for those in primary care, residents of long-term care facilities suffer from multiple chronic and debilitating illnesses that require multiple disciplines to manage. Clearly, interdisciplinary care is the ideal and, arguably, should be the standard (Zeiss & Steffen, 1996). The competent geropsychologist recognizes the unique challenges of consultation in long-term care settings as they relate to teams. First, as in other settings, the competent geropsychologist is aware of other team members and the roles they play with patients and within the team, as well as what resources are available within the facility and in consultation to the facility.

Second, while being acutely aware that confidentiality is imperative for psychologists working with teams in all settings, the fact that the team is also operating in the patient's home adds another level of sensitivity. The psychologist must be aware that any information shared with the team may be discussed by other team members in the patient's "living room" and overheard by "neighbors." While providing service in the patient's home presents some challenges, it also presents opportunities for incorporating additional members into the team, including nursing assistants, food service and housekeeping staff, and, when appropriate with patient consent, other residents.

Third, long-term care treatment teams are often more segmented than in other settings, and psychologists may have direct contact with only one segment at a time (Ogland-Hand & Zeiss, 2000). The psychologist may receive a referral from the physician, then discuss behavior issues with nursing staff, then contact family for additional information, then see the patient, followed by consultation with the nutritionist to monitor dietary intake. Developing relationships with team members in this setting is key for psychologists to maintain consistent communication and obtain all relevant information to best treat the patient.

ACUTE PHYSICAL REHABILITATION

The team model in acute rehabilitation settings began after World War II, when physicians recognized that combat survivors with severe disabilities (new to the health care community due to medical advances) could not be treated by a single discipline (Strasser et al., 2008). While there is agreement that team treatment is the only way to effectively treat these complex patients, rehabilitation teams vary widely in structure, process, and operations, and there is as yet no consensus on the effective components of a rehabilitation team (Smits et al., 2003). Teams in this setting typically include professionals from medicine, nursing, physical therapy, occupational therapy, speech therapy, psychology, recreational therapy, and social work. The role of the psychologist in rehabilitation teams varies depending on the team, the patient population (i.e., young spinal cord injury survivors versus older stroke survivors), and the training of the psychologist (rehabilitation, geriatric, and/or neuropsychology specialty). Contributions may include psychological and cognitive assessment; health interventions for pain, insomnia, and other health issues; psychotherapy for depression, anxiety, adjustment to illness, shifting roles with new onset functional deficits; and behavior management plans for disruptive behavior, among others.

In addition to previously addressed competencies, the geropsychologist in a rehabilitation setting is particularly aware of team attitudes about aging, as goals for functional status can be significantly impacted by ageist stereotypes. Issues of autonomy versus paternalism in discharge planning are commonly faced by rehabilitation teams; the psychologist acts as an advocate for the patient to assure the highest level of autonomy possible in a safe environment. The competent geropsychologist also attends to the impact of role shifts and assesses for grief in patients and families as a result of acute and chronic functional deficits.

Future Directions

Competent geropsychologists are aware of the scope of their expertise and seek training to fill needed gaps in their knowledge and skills (Knight et al., 2009). Most health care providers, including psychologists, do not get focused training in interdisciplinary teamwork, but training programs are increasingly available. The John A. Hartford Foundation developed the

Geriatrics Interdisciplinary Team Training model to facilitate interdisciplinary education about working with older adults (Fulmer, Flaherty, & Hyer, 2003). Initially targeted at physicians, nurses, and social workers, these training programs have included the full spectrum of health care providers, including psychologists. Area Health Education Centers (AHEC) along with the Veteran's Administration Interdisciplinary Team Training in Geriatrics (ITTG) and Geriatric Education Centers (GEC) are also examples of bringing students from multiple disciplines together to learn about care from an interdisciplinary perspective for older adults. While these programs are exceptional, interdisciplinary education needs to become the standard, both so that students are prepared to work in existing teams and to create a health care workforce whose focus is on collaborative care from the beginning of their careers. The future of interdisciplinary team training may also involve technology, such as online training programs (Macdonald, Stodel, & Chambers, 2008).

While the body of evidence supporting interdisciplinary teamwork in primary care is growing rapidly, there is a need for research in other settings as well. Increasing evidence-based interdisciplinary care for the most vulnerable older adults in long-term care settings is essential. Similarly, the development and evaluation of interdisciplinary efforts geared toward prevention and wellness could improve health care for older adults. Psychologists have the opportunity to play an important role in designing, implementing, and evaluating these models.

Conclusions

Interdisciplinary teamwork can significantly improve health care for older adults, particularly in treating those with multiple complex, chronic illnesses. Though "by definition, no single person can make a group become an interdisciplinary team" (Zeiss & Steffen, 1996), psychologists can enthusiastically advocate for the development and maintenance of interdisciplinary teams. To be effective members of the interdisciplinary team, psychologists should achieve competency in knowledge about models of interdisciplinary care across patient populations and settings, and in collaboration with team members maximize team functioning and provide integrated care for older adults.

PART III

Attitude Competencies

EIGHT

Individual and Cultural Diversity Considerations in Geropsychology

Yvette N. Tazeau

Americans age 65 and over now number approximately 35 million in the United States, of whom 7 million are ethnic/racial minorities (U.S. Census Bureau, 2007). These same demographic trends predict increased growth rates for minority elders as compared to White older Americans (Administration on Aging, 2008). Although these figures highlight the increasing ethnic and racial diversity among older Americans, diversity is a broader concept when considered at the individual and cultural levels. Diversity encompasses ethnicity and race as well as age, gender, income, education, location of residence, national origin (U.S.-born, foreign-born, immigrant status), language, family composition, disability (physical, cognitive, emotional), religion/spirituality, and sexual orientation. Expanding our conceptualization of geropsychology to encompass diversity as a foundational competence provides for the ability to meet the needs of today's changing demographic, of committing the profession to social responsibility, and of ensuring that core practices of assessment, intervention, and consultation will remain innovative and relevant for the needs of older adults.

Cultural competence is an ethical practice for psychology, and Behnke (2009) makes the ethical argument for valuing diversity within general psychology,

> Diversity is an ethical issue not solely because the Ethics Code requires that psychologists attend to individual differences, not solely because neglecting diversity represents an impermissible bias under the code, not solely because ignoring the role of culture and

ethnicity leaves psychologists with a poor scientific foundation for our work. Diversity is an ethical issue because we enhance the dignity and worth of the individuals and groups with whom we work when we more fully recognize, respect, and appreciate the fullness of their lives and their experiences. (p. 65)

Despite the awareness of diversity within the profession, it has been argued that proponents of multicultural psychology have often left out issues of aging and that geropsychology has not sufficiently highlighted issues of diversity (Hinrichsen, 2006; Iwasaki, Tazeau, Kimmel, Baker, & McCallum, 2009). In fact, a survey of practitioners regarding their practice with older adults and their continuing education needs failed to identify multicultural competence as a topic of interest (Qualls, Segal, Norman, Niederehe, & Gallagher-Thompson, 2002). However, just as ageism is not tolerated (American Psychological Association, 2002a), neither are other forms of discrimination, prejudice, and negative behavior. Guideline 5 of the American Psychological Association's (2004) Guidelines for Psychological Practice with Older Adults states,

Psychologists strive to understand diversity in the aging process, particularly how sociocultural factors such as gender, ethnicity, socioeconomic status, sexual orientation, disability status, and urban/rural residence may influence the experience and expression of health and of psychological problems in later life. (p. 242)

Yang and Levkoff (2005) point out that few studies address the interplay of ageism and other "isms," such as racism, from the point of view of minority older adults and health care providers. In order to counter misperceptions of minority elders, the authors propose a continuum model by which ageism in minority populations is addressed on five dimensions:

- Self-perceptions of aging (positive and negative)
- Life expectancy (such as median survival rates)
- Physiological markers (e.g., blood pressure, cholesterol, body mass index levels)
- Level of frailty (including mental and physical status, self-esteem, locus of control, etc.)
- Defensive mechanisms (e.g., degree of family and community engagement, intergenerational support)

The authors' "ageism and health" continuum represents these factors as related to stereotyping in minority older adults. The tool provides a framework in which health and cultural contexts inform the intersection of ageism and racism and its consequences. The continuum reflects historical and cultural perspectives, and although the tool is proposed for researchers it can be of use to clinicians as well in understanding the relationship between ageism and health outcomes in minority older adults.

The majority of reviews of cultural diversity in psychology in general, and in ethnogerontology in particular, still tend to reflect a limiting, traditional outline of describing the main ethnic/racial groups—African American, Asian American and Pacific Islander, Latino/Hispanic, American Indian and Alaska Native, and White—often against the backdrop of competency guidelines or frameworks. A standard general psychology resource is that of Sue and Sue's (2008) multicultural counseling, and specific to older adults is the Administration on Aging's (2001) guidebook for providers, as well as its guidelines for agencies. However, other specific minority groups also have been referenced in this fashion. For instance, Kimmel, Rose, and David (2006) provide information regarding lesbian, gay, bisexual, and transgender (LGBT) aging issues, and Banks (2008) speaks to cultural competence for women with disabilities.

The U.S. demographic profile of most minorities is diverse. For example, as a group, Asians may have many cultural similarities; however, there are cultural differences between different Asian groups such as Chinese, Japanese, and Korean. When extensive lists of cultural differences by group are presented, it is not unusual for those attempting to develop or hone their cultural competence to feel overwhelmed because of a sense that all the specifics of every group must be simultaneously mastered. The emphasis on knowledge, skills, abilities, and other attributes for cultural competence notwithstanding, at least one researcher has argued that specifically for health education for older, diverse adults there may be more utility in considering their similarities across groups (Haber, 2005).

A survey of professional psychologists regarding the use of multicultural psychotherapy competencies found that guidelines and codes carried least weight, compared to their personal and professional experiences, in influencing their development of competence regarding multicultural issues (Hansen et al., 2006). Clearly, competency guidelines, including cultural diversity ones, can benefit from a clear link to practices, and best practices and general benchmarking can be useful in this regard. But because detailing the myriad cultural aspects of all minority older adult groups clearly exceeds the scope of this chapter and potentially reduces the practical application of such knowledge for geropsychologists, the objective here is to reference contemporary cultural competency guidelines but, more important, to suggest ways in which they can be broadly mapped and applied to the practice of working with older adults across the general areas of assessment, intervention, and consultation.

Although personal experience may trump the use of competency models for some professionals, competency models do serve a very important role in providing a framework by which to learn and use specific knowledge, skills, abilities, and other attributes and characteristics regarding work with specific populations. Competency models can also provide the foundation for the development of core courses, core curriculum, and measurement of competence in individuals over time, such as through training programs. Professional geropsychology has put forth the Pikes Peak Model for training, which outlines the competencies that psychologists need to develop when working with older adults (Knight, Karel, Hinrichsen, Qualls, & Duffy, 2009). In training and service delivery, the integration of diversity competence in geropsychology can provide opportunities for a skilled workforce and thereby culturally competent, client-centered care. Increasingly, accreditation standards for training programs, hospitals, and treatment agencies seek to promote, facilitate, and advance the provision of cultural competency at all levels of care—individual, group/work team, organizational, and system (Administration on Aging, 2008; U.S. Department of Health and Human Services, 2001). Indeed, a strategy for enhancing provider effectiveness in working with culturally diverse clients is training in cultural competence (Beach et al., 2005).

Cultural or multicultural competence has been defined in various ways (Hansen, Pepitone-Arreola-Rockwell, & Greene, 2000), and because the construct has been based on different models, a singular definition accepted by all has yet to be produced. However, perhaps the most succinct definition is that of Stuart (2004): "Multicultural competence can be defined as the ability to understand and constructively relate to the uniqueness of each client in light of the diverse cultures that influence each person's perspectives" (p. 3). Within psychology, there exists a rich history of a multicultural movement (Arredondo & Perez, 2006). Competencies have been put forth by counseling psychology (Sue, Arredondo, & McDavis, 1992) and the profession as a whole (APA, 2003). An early compendium of competencies for working with older adults was provided for gerontological counseling (Myers & Schwiebert, 1996). References have been made to issues of concern in the delivery of services to minority older adults and other special populations (American Psychological Association, 1997), and more recently, competencies in the form of knowledge and skills for geropsychology have also been outlined (Molinari et al., 2003). In 2007, an APA

Council on Aging (CONA) Working Group on Multicultural Competency in Geropsychology was formed to begin to address multicultural competencies in geropsychology (APA, 2009). The effort is a preliminary step toward fully establishing multicultural competencies given that its emphasis is still mainly on ageism in general as opposed to cultural diversity concerns in particular, and its recommendations generally echo those of existing position papers for nonminority older adults.

Health Disparities

The call to extend psychology's cultural competence in addressing social inequalities, including health disparities, came almost a decade ago (Mays, 2000) and has been extended to minority elders regarding gerodiversity and social justice (Iwasaki et al., 2009):

> The term *gerodiversity* represents an approach to the issues of aging embedded within a cultural diversity framework; a framework that treats people not just as individuals but as existing within an ecological context that includes their cultural identity, cultural heritage, local social culture, family and interpersonal relationships, as well as the larger society's dominant social frameworks. (p. 72)

The authors state that the process of aging takes place within a cultural context and that clinical work with elders from different cultural backgrounds who may experience forms of discrimination or oppression implies that a social justice perspective must be considered. Health disparities, a form of social injustice, exist when underrepresented groups have reduced access to health care and receive a poorer quality of care. Minority elders have disproportionately unfavorable health outcomes regarding death, disease, and disability (Agency for Healthcare Research and Quality, 2002). Minority clients have unmet health needs based on different incidence, prevalence, and outcomes for diseases within their groups. They also experience different degrees of availability, accessibility, and barriers to services, along with different utilization rates of services.

The ways that health behaviors and the social environment contribute to health differences between and among groups have received increased attention over the years. Different minority groups experience different rates of chronic diseases such as diabetes, hypertension, and dementia. Differences are also noted in their socioeconomic status, social networks, use of and access to social support, and use of medical care. For dementia, Yeo and Gallagher-Thompson (2006) provide a robust compendium of the epidemiology of the disease for various ethnically diverse populations as well as culturally congruent methods of assessment and working with families.

For minority racial and ethnic clients, a major contributor to health disparities is a lack of culturally competent care (Institute of Medicine, 2002). An influential report describing the problems of health care that contribute to health disparities (Committee on Quality Health Care in America, 2001) stimulated the development to improve the cultural competence and cultural sensitivity of the health care environment. In fact, medical providers consider increased cultural competence as a strategy to reduce the documented disparities seen in ethnically diverse older adults for health and health care (Krisberg, 2005; Xakellis et al., 2004). A key factor in the promotion of cultural diversity considerations, and toward reduced disparities, has been the awareness that communication and language be patient-centered, family-centered, and culture-centered and that service delivery reflect an awareness of the different cultural practices, beliefs, and values. An important aspect of cultural competence is language. Approximately 49.6 million Americans speak a language other than English at home and 23.3 million have limited English proficiency (Flores, 2006). For example, 72% of first-generation Latino immigrants are primarily Spanish-speaking, and 46% of Hispanics report English as their primary language (Pew Hispanic Center, 2004). Service provider agencies that demonstrate multilingual proficiency in communicating with clients and their families are those with bilingual staff, qualified interpreters, translation services, and appropriately translated documents.

Stuart (2004) developed a dozen practical and pertinent suggestions that can facilitate incorporating a culturally competent approach to working with clients and which can apply to all aspects of assessment, intervention, and consultation with older adults. When mapped onto the framework of knowledge, skills, abilities, and other attributes, Stuart's (2004) suggestions indicate that the provider's knowledge base should reflect knowing how to determine whether the client accepts relevant cultural themes—that is, to what degree the client accepts cultural beliefs of his or her peer group—and knowing how to consider the client's worldview when selecting treatment paths including selection of other health providers, goals for treatment, and interventions.

When mapping Stuart's (2004) suggestions from a skills perspective, a skill to be developed is that of uncovering the client's unique cultural outlook. Just as important is the cultivation of sensitivity—but not an overemphasis on cultural differences—and the separation of theory from culture.

Regarding the latter, the author suggests that psychologists may make attributions about a particular cultural group based on theoretical models of how a group functions, but it is important to recognize that there are individual differences that can inform an individual group member's behavior wherein culture serves as a moderating and not causal variable. La Roche and Maxie (2003) provide 10 clinical considerations regarding how to discuss cultural differences with clients. The authors indicate that the key is having a means by which to determine how important minority identity is for the client.

Regarding abilities, a mapping of Stuart's (2004) suggestions indicates that the capacity to maintain a complex set of cultural categories in mind is important, for it allows one to be more descriptive as opposed to categorically based when understanding a client's identity. Providers also need to be able to critically evaluate how culturally relevant data are collected prior to their application to services. Knowledge of the validity and applicability of assessment measures (e.g., tests, surveys, checklists, questionnaires, and other instruments) to specific groups illustrates this suggestion. It is important to develop the ability to contextualize assessments by being able to match procedures, such as psychological tests, to the client's characteristics.

Other personal characteristics would include Stuart's (2004) suggestion of explaining one's worldview and its source, as well as its validity, in order to recognize and control personal biases (including stereotypes and prejudices). Knowing one's own values and assumptions as related to life experiences can safeguard against the imposition of a worldview on the client. Demonstrating respect for the client's beliefs and being open to changing approaches when necessary are integral to a culturally competent approach of work with clients.

Assessment

Often, some form of assessment such as phone screening, diagnostic clinical interview, or psychological testing is a point of entry for clients for health care services. The American Psychological Association's Task Force on Assessment of Competence in Professional Psychology (2006) lists as Principle 11, "The Assessment of Competence Must be Sensitive to and Highlight the Importance of Individual and Cultural Diversity" (p. 446). In the assessment process, the infusion of cultural competence comes at the intake point which allows for the cultural formulation of the older adult's background and cultural context. Ecological and cultural contexts influence the client's and the clinician's attitudes, behaviors, experiences, and views of the world. The degree to which cultural sensitivity can be made evident at the start of a client's participation in the health care system can help determine the degree to which client engagement and satisfaction are achieved.

Cultural sensitivity for many ethnic and racial minority older adults includes consideration of extended family members in the assessment process. Extended family members who serve as caregivers to the older adult can often provide important information regarding the client's status and involving them represents an integrative approach to such collateral information. Yarry, Stevens, and McCallum (2007) describe how ethnic minority older adults, as compared to older European Americans, are more likely to be part of a larger extended family context. They also describe how ethnic minority caregivers have different coping mechanisms as compared to European Americans. To account for these and other types of differences, a useful tool was developed by Ecklund and Johnson (2007), which outlines the four ingredients of a culturally competent client formulation: an intake that assesses cultural identity, cultural explanations of preexisting concerns, cultural factors related to psychosocial environment and level of functioning, and cultural elements of the relationship between the individual and the clinician. Through all of the aforementioned, migration patterns, acculturation, dialect and language, gender roles, and kinship supports and ties can be addressed by explicitly interspersing cultural questions in the interview.

Providing culturally diverse clients with a strong rationale for the assessment can help overcome potential fears of mistrust of the process. Similarly, procedures that are explained in a way that the client can understand can help dissipate any potential apprehensions. For non-English-speaking clients, the availability of multilingual staff or translators and interpreters for the diagnostic interview is critical. For psychological testing, the selection of tests, administration, scoring, interpretation, and provision of feedback should all be done within a cultural context for minority clients that considers the client's degree of familiarity and comfort with the testing process. Regarding diagnostic considerations, the prevalence of disorders among minority groups needs to be known to the provider. Practical considerations that can help put clients at ease if they have never experienced an assessment include considering a client's transportation needs, having waiting areas and other public spaces that provide displays and printed material accessible to the client and relevant to the client's culture, and ensuring that language and communication issues are addressed primarily by multilingual staff, and translators/interpreters when multilingual staff are not available.

Intervention

Pedrotti, Edwards, and Lopez (2008) make the point that individuals within the diverse U. S. population increasingly identify themselves as multiracial and suggest that strengths-based and solution-focused perspectives in psychotherapy provide contextual links for the client, a sense of belonging, and empowerment. These frameworks allow the client to be "expert" about himself or herself and in terms of culture. Clinicians familiar with the increasing use of evidence-based treatments should also be familiar with the concerns about whether and how such treatments are to be culturally adapted. Lau (2006) provides selective and directed ways in which this can be accomplished. An example of adapted treatments is the work of Gallagher-Thompson et al. (2003) for ethnically diverse caregivers of individuals with Alzheimer's disease. She and her colleagues describe how they tailored existing treatments for African American, Cuban American, and Mexican American populations to help reduce caregiver burden. Regarding multicultural competence for psychotherapy, Hansen et al. (2006) recommended that psychologists intent on developing multicultural competence recognize that it requires active effort and extra-session work; personal qualities such as perseverance and dedication to improving skills; and identification of personal barriers, including any anxieties or uncertainties about working with multicultural clients. Daniel, Roysircar, Abeles, and Boyd (2004) have also outlined individual and cultural diversity competencies for therapists.

Knowledge of the various cultural groups' health-related beliefs, cultural values, and traditional or folk healing practices of intervention is important as it may reveal a culturally diverse client's use of alternative healing and alternative medicine providers. For many ethnic minority groups these beliefs also dovetail with religious and spiritual practices. Religiosity is often used as a coping mechanism for illness and is related to health and well-being (Klemmack et al., 2007; Park, 2007). A study (The National Quality Forum, 2006, pp. 36–38) found that up to 77% of patients would like spiritual/religious issues considered as part of their medical care, yet only 10% to 20% of care providers discussed the issues with their patients. Religious participation, religious coping, and spirituality have been found to be higher among African Americans and Caribbean Blacks as compared to older Whites (Taylor, Chatters, & Jackson, 2007).

Older Latinos living in Latin America or the Caribbean who reported high religious affiliation also reported better self-rated health (Reyes-Ortiz, Palaez, Koenig, & Mulligan, 2007). A useful tool for this important cultural dimension was developed by Nelson-Becker and Nakashima (2007), wherein 11 domains in spirituality are identified that can be assessed when working with older adults.

Other forms of intervention for older adults include behavioral health interventions, pharmacological interventions, and knowledge of and referral to appropriate community resources for minority groups. Knowledge of incidence and prevalence rates of disorders among the different minority groups is as important for intervention as for assessment. Similarly, familiarity regarding differential aspects of pharmacological interventions in minority elderly is also important for treatment planning. Some minority elders may have culturally based suspicions regarding the use of medication as they prefer natural healing methods and may forgo taking their prescription medications, or take them in combination with naturopathic treatments.

Consultation

Geropsychologists are frequently called upon to interact and collaborate with other health care service providers in different forms of teams, be they integrative, interdisciplinary, intradisciplinary, or transdisciplinary. Culturally competent geropsychologists can bring their strength to such teams regarding conceptualizing cases contextually, that is, embracing a reliance on a patient-centered, culturally sensitive approach to health care (Herman et al., 2007). Psychologists interface with other disciplines, and through their role on teams they can communicate and advocate regarding prevention, program development, or crisis intervention as well as build partnerships and policies. Geropsychologists also coordinate care such as transitions of clients back to home, provide support for palliative care, and consult regarding end-of-life concerns. Ethnic minority older adults, such as Latinos and Koreans, for example, fit in more with family-centered models of care regarding decisions about long-term care and terminal conditions (Blackhall et al., 1995).

Individual geropsychologists alone cannot be sole purveyors of cultural competence; the agencies where they work must also embrace an organizational culture that reflects cultural competence for its clients. The degree to which an agency promotes diversity throughout the organization in hiring, retention, and promotion of diverse staff is a key factor in the agency's ability to provide culturally diverse services. Reese, Melton, and

Ciaravino's (2004) study of hospice and palliative care directors found that culturally diverse groups were not gaining greater access to end-of-life care, and it appears that what makes the difference is higher recruitment levels of more diverse volunteers in the programs. The presence of the volunteers predicted a more diverse patient population. In a study of hospice workers and volunteers, Schim, Doorenbos, and Borse (2006) found that educational interventions enhanced their cultural competence. The training workshops focused on the concepts of cultural diversity, knowledge, awareness, and competence behaviors. Goode and Sockalingam (2000) report that the National Center for Cultural Competence (NCCC) developed a definition, checklist, and cogent reasons for incorporating cultural competence into home health organizational policy. These studies notwithstanding, Curtis and Dreachslin's (2008) review of the literature on diversity management from 2000 to 2005 yielded few studies examining the effectiveness of specific diversity interventions in organizations and provided limited guidance regarding the design and implementation of diversity interventions. Psychologists can play an important role in helping agencies reach diversity goals by gauging the degree of organizational responsiveness to culturally diverse clients, such as through the creation of rating instruments, surveys, focus groups, and other tools.

Conclusions

Geropsychology is today a practice involving interactions with older adults of various and differing individual and cultural backgrounds. For many years now, it has been documented that health and disability differences exist among ethnic and racial groups, as well as other cultural groups. Sue (2008) argues that multicultural consultation to organizations, by its very nature, has at its core a key aspect of social justice because it involves removing barriers to equal access and opportunity in organizations. Quality care has at its core equity, that is, that there be fairness and justice regarding the right to access to and ownership of quality care. When organizations serving older adults make the case for aspects such as quality, business, risk management, and accreditation and regulation, equity should also be an integral component (Massachusetts General Hospital Institute for Health Policy, 2009). Other professional disciplines with which psychology works closely, such as social work, nursing, medicine, occupational therapy, physical therapy, speech and language therapy, and pharmacy, have taken steps to help reduce health disparities through the adoption of cultural competence guidelines (Crewe, 2004; Giger et al., 2007; Xakellis et al., 2004).

Psychology knows how to assess competence (Kaslow et al., 2007); geropsychologists now have an obligation to put forth and support multicultural competencies for practice with older adults. Indeed, cultural competence was one of the main recommendations promulgated by the 2006 Pikes Peak conference and outlined in the *Pikes Peak Geropsychology Knowledge and Skill Assessment Tool, Version 1.0* (Council of Professional Geropsychology Training Programs, 2008). It is time to be active and emphatically declarative promoters of cultural competence or, in the words of Nezu (2005), "culturally asseverative."

NINE

Ethics

Michele J. Karel

The ability to appreciate and apply ethical and legal standards is a foundational competency for professional psychology practice (Rodolfa et al., 2005), one of the "building blocks" underlying everything we do as professional psychologists. Like all psychology practice, professional geropsychology practice is guided by the *Ethical Principles of Psychologists and Code of Conduct* (American Psychological Association, 2002b). The core principles of the APA Ethics Code—beneficence and nonmalfeasance, fidelity and responsibility, integrity, justice, and respect for people's rights and dignity—are entirely pertinent to psychological practice with older adults.

Ethical practice with older adults, families, and related care systems entails additional and complementary knowledge and skills, due to specific clinical issues and settings of care for many older adults. According to the Pikes Peak Model competencies, a foundational competency for geropsychology practice is to understand and apply ethical and legal standards, with particular attention to aging-specific issues, such as "informed consent, confidentiality, capacity and competency, end-of-life decision making, and elder abuse and neglect" (Knight, Karel, Hinrichsen, Qualls, & Duffy, 2009, p. 208).

Special ethical and legal considerations in serving older populations are influenced by the following:

1. A significant minority of older adults have compromised decision-making capacity related to dementia or other neuropsychiatric disorders, raising frequent questions about how best to make decisions with or for these elders (Moye & Marson, 2007; Qualls & Smyer, 2007).

2. Interdisciplinary collaboration is often fundamental to excellent geriatric care, but this model of care can also raise challenging dilemmas regarding confidentiality and team decision making (Mezey et al., 2002).

3. Older adults are often embedded in the social context of their family systems; family members are frequently involved as caregivers, advocates, or spokespersons with or for the older adult, which can also raise questions about confidentiality and appropriate locus of decision making (Karel & Moye, 2006; Qualls, 1999).

4. Older adults who receive psychological services in inpatient medical, rehabilitation, or long-term care settings may face real constraints on privacy and self-determination (e.g., many rules, or limited choices, in an institutional care environment; Karel, 2008).

5. Physically, cognitively, or psychiatrically frail older adults are more vulnerable to physical and psychological abuse or neglect, as well as financial exploitation (National Center on Elder Abuse, www.ncea.aoa.gov).

6. Older adults are more likely to die than younger adults, and often face difficult decisions about care at the end of life (Hawkins, Ditto, Danks, & Smucker, 2005; Winzelberg, Hanson, & Tulsky, 2005).

7. The aging population is increasingly diverse in terms of cultural background, country of birth, and native language (Federal Interagency Forum on Aging-Related Statistics, 2008). Important cultural differences exist regarding meanings of and norms for aging, illness, caregiving, utilization of health care services, medical decision making, death and dying, and so forth; thus all ethical challenges must be considered in cultural context (American Geriatrics Society, 2004; Karel, 2007a; Xakellis et al., 2004).

This chapter has three broad aims. First, there is a detailed review of the foundational competencies for ethical geropsychology practice, including the fundamental tension between the values of respecting the autonomy versus protecting the safety of an older adult; the concept of decision making capacity; the challenges of surrogate decision making; and legal, clinical, and social tools central to working with vulnerable older adults.

Second, specific ethical issues that can arise in psychological assessment, intervention, consultation, and research with older adults or care systems are identified. And finally, a model for ethical decision making in geriatric care is presented.

Ethical and Legal Standards: Foundational Competencies for Geropsychology Practice

In an effort to develop a geropsychology competency evaluation tool, each Pikes Peak knowledge and skill competency was broken down into further detailed abilities (Karel, Emery, & Molinari, in press) The foundational geropsychology competency addressing ethical and legal standards was broken down into four specific abilities. Competent geropsychologists are able to

> identify complex ethical and legal issues that arise in the care of older adults, analyze them accurately, and proactively address them, including: (a) tension between sometimes competing goals of promoting autonomy and protecting safety of at-risk older adults; (b) decision making capacity and strategies for optimizing older adults' participation in informed consent regarding a wide range of medical, residential, financial, and other life decisions; (c) surrogate decision making as indicated regarding a wide range of medical, residential, financial, end of life, and other life decisions; and (d) state and organizational laws and policies covering elder abuse, advance directives, conservatorship, guardianship, multiple relationships, and confidentiality (see http://www.uccs.edu/~cpgtp/).

Foundational competence in ethical geropsychology practice is closely related to other foundational competencies, including collaborating with interdisciplinary teams, addressing individual and cultural diversity, practicing self-reflection, and implementing appropriate geropsychology business practices. These building blocks of professional geropsychology practice are, of necessity, intertwined and will be addressed, as appropriate, in this review about foundational ethical competence. Further, the ability to identify and analyze ethical dilemmas will be addressed in the concluding section of this chapter.

PROMOTING AUTONOMY AND PROTECTING SAFETY

Two fundamental values underlying ethics in Western medical practice and professional psychology include respect for individual autonomy—that individuals have the right to decide what is best for themselves, consistent with their values and beliefs—and beneficence, that is, the intent to do good, and do no harm, on behalf of a patient (American Psychological Association, 2002b; Beauchamp & Childress, 2001; Mueller, Hook, & Fleming, 2004). Most often, the principles of autonomy and beneficence coincide to help guide a plan of care; usually patients and health care providers agree, after education and discussion, about the best course of action for the patient.

However, what a patient wants and what a health care professional, team, or family member thinks is best often do not coincide. Sometimes, older adults are not interested in further medical or surgical interventions ("leave me alone, I've had enough"). Or, older adults have different notions about their health and safety than others do. For example, family members may question an older person's ability to live alone safely, drive, or manage her bank account, while the older person insists she is fine. Or, if in an institutional setting, a patient has repeated falls or wanders off the unit, to what extent should the patient's freedom be restricted to ensure her safety? People with intact decision-making capacity have the right to make risky, eccentric, or otherwise unpopular decisions, as long as they do not put others at risk. However, people who have difficulty understanding and appreciating the risks and benefits inherent in a situation need assistance negotiating that difficult balance between doing what one wants and doing what is best (the latter is usually open to varying interpretations).

The types of life decisions that are relevant in terms of supporting older adults' autonomy and protecting their safety range from simple everyday choices to life and death decisions. Geropsychologists are familiar with the range of life domains and decisions that older adults, family members, and health care professionals encounter. Broadly speaking, decisions (and related functional capacities), may fall into one of the following six categories (American Bar Association and American Psychological Association Assessment of Capacity in Older Adults Project Working Group, 2008):

1. Medical decision making (Moye, Gurrera, Karel, Edelstein, & O'Connell, 2006)—for example, from making simple decisions about medications through decisions about care at the end of life (Karlawish, Quill, & Meier, 1999)

2. Financial management (Marson, 2001; Marson & Hebert, 2005) — from paying one's bills through managing complex investments

3. Independent living (Moye & Braun, 2007), regarding the degree of independence versus supervision needed in one's residential setting

4. Driving—if and when an older adult may drive safely (Bieliauskas, 2005; Veterans Health Administration National Ethics Committee, 2007b; Wild & Cotrell, 2003)

5. Relationships and sexuality—for example, to what degree may older adults with cognitive impairment select their sexual partners (Lyden, 2007; Marson & Huthwaite, 2005)

6. Testamentary capacity, or the ability to make a will (Marson & Hebert, 2005).

In addition, decisions to participate in research studies are particularly important, especially regarding protecting potentially vulnerable elders (Alzheimer's Association, 2004; Kim, Appelbaum, Jeste, & Olin, 2004; Kim, Caine, Currier, Leibovici, & Ryan, 2001).

The great majority of older adults remain perfectly capable of making decisions for themselves or deciding that they prefer others to help them make decisions. Ageist attitudes can, at times, lead well-intentioned people to assume that an older adult can not fully understand or make decisions for herself. We must all confront such possibly ageist attitudes in ourselves and really listen to, know, and respect the older adults we work with. The older adults who raise concerns about autonomy versus safety are those who do have compromised insight and judgment related to symptoms of dementia, psychiatric disorders (e.g., delusional disorder, severe depression), severe personality disorders, or complicated medical issues. In cases of obviously and severely impaired elders (e.g., advanced dementia with minimal capacity for communication), it is clear that surrogate decision makers must do what they can to protect the well-being of the individual, consistent with the known values of that person to the extent possible. However, a minority of older adults who remain clearly able to express their preferences might be characterized as having marginal capacity, perhaps in the early stages of a progressive dementia, because they have increased difficulty appreciating the risks inherent in some situations.

Among older adults and their family members, and among geriatric care professionals, individuals vary considerably in the extent to which they emphasize the goals of promoting autonomy versus protecting safety, and in the extent to which they are willing or able to tolerate risk (Kane & Caplan, 1990; Mezey et al., 2002). Important professional, cultural, institutional/agency, family system, and personality differences influence relative values for autonomy promotion versus safety protection, and this tension leads to many of the ethical dilemmas in geriatric care. Professionals on the same health care team may differ in their views on what is best for a particular patient (Burck & Lapidos, 2002; Chichin & Mezey, 2002). Likewise, patients and different family members may have conflicting views, and views that are not in agreement with those of various health care team members. It is important to realize that nobody is "right or wrong" in these situations; there is simply a disagreement between different honored ethical principles or values and, usually, well-intentioned people.

Geropsychologists appreciate that professionals from other disciplines are trained and socialized into different cultures of care. Physicians, nurses, social workers, psychologists, rehabilitation therapists, and other geriatric team members often have differing ideas about issues such as locus of responsibility for decision making, extent to which the patient and/or family are considered part of the team, the scope of assessment and treatment options, extent to which protecting a patient's safety versus facilitating autonomy is prioritized, and what range of outcomes is considered "good" (Burck & Lapidos, 2002; Nelson, Allen, & Cox., 2005; Qualls & Czirr, 1988). Further, all health care professionals come from their own individual cultural, religious, and family background and may view responses to aging patients differently through those lenses as well. Let's look at the following case example.

Mr. Sanders is a 78-year-old, widowed Irish American who lives alone in his house where he has lived for 40+ years. He enjoys his privacy and working in the garden. He has lived independently and safely in the 10 years since his wife died. One son lives an hour's drive away, and one daughter lives in a distant state and visits several times each year. Mr. Sanders's children have noticed that he's not as steady on his feet, and that he seems more forgetful in recent months. One day, he fell when bringing tools up from the basement and fractured his leg. Fortunately, he was able to make his way to the phone and called 911. He was admitted to the hospital, and then to a rehabilitation unit for physical therapy and, after 2 months, was able to walk using a cane. A team meeting was held to discuss discharge planning: Mr. Sanders' daughter flew in and his son was there too. Mr. Sanders clearly wanted to return home. His daughter didn't think that was a good idea. His son was not sure, but wanted to respect his father's wishes. The physician thought he'd be better off in an assisted living facility. The social worker thought he could institute a trial to return home with some services, including a life line alert and increased help from his kids to manage his finances and medications, as well as a promise that he would not try to negotiate the stairs to the basement.

DECISION-MAKING CAPACITY AND OPTIMIZING OLDER
ADULTS' PARTICIPATION IN DECISION MAKING

In ethics case consultations, one of the important clarifying questions often is, "Who has the right to make the decision here?" If the patient is considered to have intact decision-making capacity, then ultimately he or she gets to make the decision as long as it is within the constraints of the law and institutional policies, and does not impose unfair demands on others. For example, if Mr. Sanders is able to understand the risks and benefits of returning home and can clearly express the reasons for his choice, then one might say that he has the capacity to decide to continue to live in his own home, despite possible risks. If a patient does not have the capacity to make a particular decision (e.g., about medical care, finances, residential choices), then a surrogate decision maker must be identified (see next section). Therefore, much hinges on this concept of decision-making capacity: What is it? How do we evaluate it? How would we know if Mr. Sanders really has the capacity to make an informed decision about living alone in his suburban home?

Decision-making capacity is a conceptually complex construct. In legal contexts, it is an all-or-nothing judgment: An individual either has or lacks a particular capacity (e.g., for financial management). Historically, this legal determination of capacity has been known more frequently by the term *competency*. Even in clinical settings, staff often speak of capacity in black and white terms, "Oh, he's not competent," based on a subjective impression of the patient's behavior or attitude. However, in clinical reality, capacity is best thought of as existing along a continuum, with full capacity and incapacity anchoring the ends of a continuum, with a range of "diminished capacities" in between. In terms of distinguishing between legal determinations versus clinical opinions, it can help to use the terms *legal capacity* versus *clinical capacity* (American Bar Association and American Psychological Association Assessment of Capacity in Older Adults Project Working Group, 2008).

Further, capacity is domain specific. For example, a person may need help with finances but be able to make health care decisions. Even within the financial domain, a person may maintain capacity to manage a simple checking account but not to manage multiple investments or accounts. Capacity is also context dependent. A person may maintain the capacity to live alone in an urban apartment with easy access to groceries, medical care, and help from neighbors, but be unable to live safely in a large house in the suburbs with few supports or transportation options. Capacity may also change over time. For example, during an acute illness, mental status changes may adversely affect a person's decision-making capacity, which may return to baseline capacity after recovery. Alternatively, such as in the case of progressive dementia, capacities are expected to deteriorate over time (American Bar Association and American Psychological Association Assessment of Capacity in Older Adults Project Working Group, 2008; Ganzini, Volicer, Nelson, & Derse 2003; Moye, 2007).

Psychologists, other health care providers, attorneys, and judges need to appreciate emerging models for capacity assessment if they are to protect the rights and safety of vulnerable older adults (American Bar Association and American Psychological Association Assessment of Capacity in Older Adults Project Working Group, 2005, 2006, 2008; Moye, Butz, Marson, & Wood, 2007; Moye, 2007; Moye & Marson, 2007). Historically, assessments of capacity have been fairly subjective and unreliable (Marson, McInturff, Hawkins, Bartolucci, & Harrell, 1997). Research over the past 2 decades has helped to clarify concepts, models, and measurement of capacity (Moye, Butz, et al., 2007; Moye et al., 2006; Qualls & Smyer, 2007). Clinical judgments about capacity should be based upon an understanding of how underlying diagnoses that affect cognitive and/or emotional functioning (important to specify how) influence everyday functioning in domains of concern (e.g., ability to do activities of daily living, to make medical decisions, to drive). Additionally, clinical capacity judgments reflect an appreciation of the values and preferences of the older adult, the risk of harm and extent of supervision needed, and means to optimize the person's functioning. Such models are helping to influence guardianship reform (Moye, Butz, et al., 2007; Moye, Wood, et al., 2007; see Edelstein and Koven's chapter, "Older Adult Assessment Issues and Strategies," in this volume for more information on capacity evaluation and related assessment tools).

Professional geropsychologists are informed about concepts of decisional and functional capacity, and they work to clarify and optimize capacities of their clients. Many well-intentioned people tend to "take over" decision making or functioning for older adults with diminished capacity, when many of these elders are still well able to participate in making decisions about their life, if they wish to. People with mild to moderate dementia are able to communicate their values, beliefs, and preferences (Carpenter, Kissel, & Lee., 2007; Feinberg & Whitlatch, 2001; Karel, Moye, Bank, & Azar, 2007; Whitlatch, Feinberg, & Tucke, 2005). Many things can be done to optimize an older adult's decision-making participation, such as addressing the person's sensory deficits, reducing distractions, using visual and memory aids, asking questions simply and clearly, and demonstrating clear respect for the older adult's input. Likewise, it is important to respect cultural and personality differences in the extent to which older adults want to make their own decisions or defer to the judgments of family members, health care professionals, clergy, or others (Karel, 2007a; Xakellis et al., 2004).

One important way of optimizing an older adult's autonomy is to be aware of and encourage the process of advance care planning. This process allows older adults who currently maintain decision-making capacities to plan ahead for a time when their abilities may be compromised (discussed in a later section). Even older adults with some degree of cognitive impairment are well able to name people they trust to speak for them in times of incapacity (Mezey, Teresi, Ramsey, Mitty, & Bobrowitz, 2000) and to express values and preferences related to everyday living and medical decisions (Carpenter et al., 2007; Karel, Moye, et al., 2007). Let's return to the example of Mr. Sanders.

In the case of Mr. Sanders, the rehabilitation team asked the psychologist to evaluate his capacity to make a decision regarding discharge planning. In addition, the physical therapist (PT) and occupational therapist (OT) provided their opinions about his functional abilities. The PT and OT felt that he could negotiate most situations independently, and that he remained able to complete his own activities of daily living and most instrumental activities of daily living. However, the OT felt that he needed some assistance organizing his pillbox and managing his bills and finances. The PT felt that he was at risk for falling if going up or down stairs without being able to hold on to a solid railing. The psychologist's evaluation suggested that Mr. Sanders had mild memory problems, and mild problems with organization and planning, but that he did understand and appreciate the risks and benefits of staying in his own home as well as the recommendations for help, and that he was thus able to make the decision on his own. Mr. Sanders decided to return home, and his son was agreeable to visiting each weekend to help Mr. Sanders with his bills and to set up his weekly pillbox. Mr. Sanders and his daughter agreed that it would help them both for her to have a nightly "check in" call with him. In addition, Mr. Sanders' family and team expressed some concern about his local driving, given his mild cognitive deficits. Mr. Sanders insisted he was fine to drive, but agreed to have a rehabilitation driving evaluation.

SURROGATE DECISION MAKING

Providing psychological services to older adults often entails working closely with informal or formal surrogate decision makers, those who take on responsibility for helping to make life decisions on behalf of the older adult. Of note, many fully capable older adults prefer a model of shared decision making, with family and/or health care providers, especially regarding decisions about end-of-life care (Puchalski et al., 2000; Rosenfeld, Wenger, & Kagawa-Singer, 2000). Further, older adults from certain cultural backgrounds prefer to defer medical decision making to their adult children or other family members (Blackhall, Murphy, Frank, & Michel, 1995; Hornung et al., 1998; Yeo & Gallagher-Thompson, 2006). We are embedded in our social contexts; promoting individual autonomy does not necessarily mean that individuals prefer to make decisions in isolation from others. Therefore, family members or friends may be involved in the care of capable older adults, simply as advocates or social supports. Several studies suggest that "companions" who join older adults for medical visits help to facilitate older adults' participation in decision making as well as patient satisfaction with physician care (Clayman, Roter, Wissow, & Bandeen-Roche, 2005; Wolff & Roter, 2008). In terms of providing psychological services, ethical challenges can arise in determining the appropriate extent of family involvement (discussed in a later section).

Surrogate decision making refers to one person being responsible for making decisions on behalf of another when that person is no longer capable to make informed decisions for herself. Sometimes a surrogate has been clearly designated by a legal mechanism, such as a durable power of attorney for health care or financial issues, or through establishment of a formal legal guardianship. More often, family caregivers assume the role of surrogate decision makers, simply as the older adult's next of kin (Karel & Moye, 2006). When it is unclear which family member should serve as the decision maker, especially in cases of conflict, guidelines usually respect next of kin in the following order: spouse, adult child, parent, sibling. However, these guidelines may not help identify the person who best knows the older adult or has the older person's best interest closest to heart. This point is particularly important for gay and lesbian elders who have a trusted partner.

For example, if Mr. Sanders is found in the future to lack decision-making capacity, his son and daughter may disagree as to the best plan of care. It would help, in this situation, for Mr. Sanders to have designated one of them as his health care proxy, indicating whom he trusts most to make decisions on his behalf. Or perhaps he most trusts his cousin, and it would help to know that. Sometimes, an ethics committee needs to be consulted when there are questions about who is the most appropriate surrogate decision maker. Often, with clear and respectful discussion, a consensus can be reached on a plan of care.

How should surrogate decision makers reach decisions on behalf of another person? While this discussion centers on health care decisions, the same questions can be raised about financial, residential, or other legal decisions that a surrogate might have to address. From an ethical perspective, surrogate decision makers are expected to use the principle of "substituted judgment" to guide decisions to the extent possible (President's Commission for the Study of Ethical Problems in Medicine and Biomedical and Behavioral Research, 1983). That is, the surrogate attempts to make the decision that the patient would have made if the patient could still speak for herself, based on knowledge of the patient's previously expressed values, beliefs, or preferences. If there is insufficient information upon which to make a substituted judgment, then surrogates are to be guided by a "best interest" standard. That is, the surrogate makes a decision that would generally be considered in the best interest of the now incompetent person.

In reality, research and practice have demonstrated that the substituted judgment standard is difficult to meet. For one, it is unclear that any individual could know with certainty what types of care she would want in a future state of physical or mental health (Koppelman, 2002). Even in the case of people who have completed a living will, stating general or specific preferences for medical care in the event of incapacity, there are challenges. While a living will can provide some guidance, it can also be difficult to know if the person's preferences definitely would be the same now as at the time the document was originally drafted (Degrazia, 1999). Moreover, it can be difficult to apply a general directive ("I don't want aggressive medical interventions to keep me alive") to a specific clinical situation. Further, multiple research studies using hypothetical scenarios have demonstrated that family members and health care providers are generally unable to predict a patient's health care preferences (Hare, Pratt, & Nelson, 1992; Suhl, Simons, Reedy, & Garrick, 1994).

A consensus-based approach, considering what is known about the patient's past and present values and priorities, along with the burdens and benefits of different treatment options, is an important model to guide surrogate decision making (Karlawish et al., 1999; Veterans Health Administration National Ethics Committee, 2007a; Volicer et al., 2002).

In many cases, the older adult is able to participate to some degree in decision making and can provide assent if not full informed consent regarding a plan of care (Molinari et al., 2004).

It is increasingly accepted that the burdens and benefits of different options for family caregivers have a legitimate place in decision making. Families have a right to consider their own health, mental health, and financial interests in making care decisions for a loved one (Veterans Health Administration National Ethics Committee, 2007a). Most older adults are, in fact, very clear that they are concerned about the interests of their families (Karel & Gatz, 1996). Surrogate decision making regarding end-of-life care can be especially stressful, and families need good education and support through this process (Haley et al., 2002; Sachs, Shega, & Cox-Hayley, 2004; Winzelberg et al., 2005), including information about options for palliative and hospice care. The Veterans Health Administration developed recommendations to help proxy decision makers develop care plans for incapacitated long-term care residents (Volicer et al., 2002).

Geropsychologists may work at times with older adults who have no next of kin or others to serve as surrogate decision makers. These cases are particularly challenging, especially when that older person clearly needs assistance and protection. In such cases, court-appointed legal guardianship is often sought. Yet, the guardian is then asked to make important decisions regarding a person few people know much about. There are models to help guide surrogate decision making for "unbefriended" elders (Gillick, 1995). Ideally, guardians do what they can to learn about the background, values, and commitments of their wards (Moye, Butz, et al., 2007; Vig et al., 2007).

CLINICAL AND LEGAL TOOLS TO PROTECT
SELF-DETERMINATION AND SAFETY OF OLDER ADULTS

Geropsychologists are aware of clinical and legal resources available to help older adults plan for potential future incapacity as well as to help protect vulnerable older adults. Advance care planning is promoted in the field of gerontology. Advance care planning is a process of communicating and documenting preferences for future care in case one is unable to make decisions for oneself in the future. In this sense, it is a process that aims to promote the autonomy of an individual in a future state of incapacity. While advance care planning typically refers to health care preferences, the process may equally apply to planning ahead for financial, residential, and other life decisions.

Therefore, in working with older adults who are healthy or who have mild signs of cognitive impairment, it is helpful to discuss options for advance care planning. In the health care realm, individuals may complete advance directives, which are typically regulated by state law. There are two major types of advance directives. The first is designation of a durable power of attorney for health care, or a health care proxy, to manage health care decision making if the older adult is considered incapable of making her own decisions. The second type is an instructional directive, often called a living will, which specifies goals of future medical care and/or specific medical interventions that would be desired or not at some future date (Fischer, Arnold, & Tulsky, 2000). Many Web sites allow download of advance directives from each state (e.g., National Hospice and Palliative Care Organization, 2007, at www.caringinfo.org; U.S. Living Will Registry, 2008, at www.uslivingwillregistry.com).

The Patient Self-Determination Act, passed in 1990, requires health care facilities that receive federal funds to inform patients of their rights to complete an advance directive. Since that time, extensive research has documented that simply completing an advance directive document does not ensure that medical care will be consistent with patients' or family's goals or preferences (Teno et al., 1997). Instead, advance care planning is a process that entails ongoing communication in the context of a patient's social network (Hammes & Rooney, 1998; Karel, Powell, & Cantor, 2004; Prendergast, 2001).

Other tools that can aid the process of advance health care planning include use of values histories to clarify, document, and communicate the values and beliefs that might guide future health care preferences (Hammes & Rooney, 1998; Karel, 2000; Karel et al., 2004; Pearlman et al., 1998; Pearlman, Starks, Cain, & Cole, 2005). Patients and families may benefit from sharing such discussions about values for health care. A number of advance care planning "toolkits" or other materials are available at Web sites, including American Bar Association Commission on Law and Aging Consumer's Tool Kit for Health Care Advance Planning, at www.abanet.org/aging/toolkit/home.html, and the National Hospice and Palliative Care Organization, www.caringinfo.org/PlanningAhead.htm. Similarly, advance proxy plans allow family members and health care teams to define the goals of care for persons with dementia when they are admitted to a long-term care setting (Cantor & Pearlman, 2004; Volicer et al., 2002). Likewise, a number of values assessment tools are available to help patients, families, and professional caregivers plan for meeting the everyday needs of individuals in long-term and home-care settings (Carpenter, Van Haitsma, Ruckdeschel, & Lawton, 2000; Whitlatch et al., 2005).

In the financial domain, older adults may designate a power of attorney, giving authority to another person (called an "agent") to manage one's financial affairs. A financial power of attorney may be crafted so that it takes place immediately, whether or not the older adult is incapacitated, or only at a time of future incapacity. A *durable* power of attorney allows the agent to retain decision making rights even after an adult becomes incapacitated. An older adult can specify that the agent has the power to handle all financial matters, or can specify or limit the agent's powers. Likewise, many adults choose to complete a will (last will and testament) to instruct survivors on management or distribution of their assets after death. Information about these legal tools is available on Web sites such as www.abanet.org, www.nolo.com, and www.aarp.org.

Other legal protections are available for adults who are already incapacitated and found unable to make decisions or to care for themselves. A guardian is a person appointed by the court to be responsible for the personal affairs of an incapacitated person (in the context of adult guardianship). Likewise, a conservator is a person appointed by a court to be responsible for the finances and assets of an incapacitated person. Guardianship law is handled by the states, and definitions of "incapacity" and processes for appointing and monitoring guardians vary considerably across localities. Recent years have seen a movement toward guardianship reform in many states given concerns about historically limited due process, overly controlling interventions, and poor accountability (Moye, Wood, et al., 2007; Wood, 2004). An important part of these reforms has been to increase the use of limited guardianship orders. That is, instead of a guardian taking over all life decisions for an adult, limited guardianships are constructed to address only the life domains for which the adult needs assistance, thereby balancing goals of protecting the older adult with maintaining as much autonomy and dignity as possible (Moye, Butz, et al., 2007; Moye, Wood, et al., 2007).

The American Bar Association Commission on Law and Aging and the American Psychological Association joined forces to form the Assessment of Capacity in Older Adults Project Working Group, with the aim of clarifying—for lawyers, judges, and psychologists—definitions and processes for evaluating the capacity of older adults. Three handbooks address this critical issue from the perspective of the professional role of lawyers (American Bar Association and American Psychological Association Assessment of Capacity in Older Adults Project Working

Group, 2005), judges (American Bar Association and American Psychological Association Assessment of Capacity in Older Adults Project Working Group, 2006), and psychologists (American Bar Association and American Psychological Association Assessment of Capacity in Older Adults Project Working Group, 2008). These three handbooks are available, free of charge, at the APA Office on Aging Web site at www.apa.org/pi/aging/. Psychologists are increasingly recognized for their expertise in capacity evaluation and, in many states, are authorized to complete guardianship certificates for the court.

Elder abuse and neglect is sadly a prevalent problem, and every state has laws and services addressing the protection of vulnerable elders (Mellor & Brownelll, 2006). The U.S. Administration on Aging established the National Center on Elder Abuse (NCEA) in 1988, to serve as a national resource center to prevent the mistreatment of older adults. The NCEA Web site is an important resource for information about elder abuse and has links to information about adult protective services in every state (www.ncea.aoa.gov). Psychologists are mandated reporters for elder abuse or neglect in most states. Geropsychologists recognize signs of elder abuse or neglect and are aware of laws regarding mandated reporting and the resources of Adult Protective Services, and elder services more generally, in their localities.

Geropsychologists are aware of other national and local resources available to aid in the protection of vulnerable elders. The U.S. Administration on Aging (AoA) "works through the national aging network of 56 State Units on Aging, 655 Area Agencies on Aging, 236 Tribal and Native organizations representing 300 American Indian and Alaska Native Tribal organizations, and two organizations serving Native Hawaiians, plus thousands of service providers, adult care centers, caregivers, and volunteers" (from the AoA Website at www.aoa.gov). The AoA Web site has links for information about a wide range of services for both professionals and for older adults and their families. Resources include legal assistance, health insurance counseling, prevention of fraud and abuse, long-term care ombudsman programs, eldercare locator services, and information and referral for family caregivers.

Finally, geropsychologists should be aware of their local and/or institutional policies regarding elder care issues, and resolution of ethical dilemmas. Many hospitals and long-term care settings have ethics advisory committees available to help with resolution of ethical dilemmas (Aulisio, Arnold, & Youngner, 2000; Hester, 2007). For older adults in long-term care facilities, each state manages a Long-Term Care Ombudsman Program that works to investigate and resolve complaints regarding care in a particular setting (Huber et al., 2001). Information about this program can also be found at the AoA Web site, www.aoa.gov.

Ethical Issues Related to Geropsychological Assessment, Intervention, Consultation, and Research

So far, this review has addressed common ethical issues that arise in geriatric care that are not necessarily specific to professional psychology practice. This section highlights ethical issues that arise in providing geropsychology assessment, intervention, and consultation services (Bush, 2008; Karel, 2008; Lichtenberg et al., 1998) as well as ethical issues pertaining to research with vulnerable older adult populations.

GEROPSYCHOLOGICAL ASSESSMENT

Geropsychologists provide a range of psychological assessment services, consistent with their own professional competencies and as relevant to the populations they serve. Geropsychological assessment may include interview-based psychodiagnostic assessment; standardized evaluations of mood, personality, or psychiatric symptomatology; cognitive evaluations; and decision making or other functional capacity evaluations. Some of these evaluations are requested to help devise an appropriate plan of care and may yield recommendations regarding the level of care or supervision needed by the older adult. The outcome of a capacity evaluation may lead to a loss of decision-making rights by the older adult. Therefore, an older adult participating in geropsychological evaluation has both a lot to gain (hopefully, access to mental health or other services that will ultimately be helpful and improve quality of life) and potentially a lot to lose (the right to make one's own decisions, moving out of one's home to a more restrictive care environment).

Geropsychologists obtain informed consent from older adults, or their surrogates, to proceed with a psychological assessment. Informed consent includes adequate disclosure of information about the purpose, procedures, and possible risks and benefits of the evaluation; communication that participation is voluntary; and a client who has the capacity to understand, appreciate, and reason through the risks and benefits of participation (Berg, Appelbaum, Lidz, & Parker, 2001). So, what happens when the purpose of the evaluation is to evaluate an older adult's decision-making capacity? Sometimes, such clients can still understand the purpose of the evaluation and provide informed consent or refusal. At other times, an older client is not able to understand the purpose of the evaluation and may either agree to proceed (i.e., provide "assent"; Molinari et al., 2004), or refuse the evaluation without really understanding the implications. In all of these cases, the outcome of the attempt to obtain informed consent must be documented. If an older adult already has an authorized surrogate decision maker (health care proxy, legal guardian), then that surrogate should provide consent to proceed with a geropsychological evaluation.

The ABA/APA handbook for psychologists, *Assessment of Older Adults with Diminished Capacity*, provides a good overview of clinical approaches for capacity evaluation, including challenges related to informed consent (American Bar Association and American Psychological Association Assessment of Capacity in Older Adults Project Working Group, 2008). The APA Ethics Code (American Psychological Association, 2002b, p. 1065) specifically states that full informed consent is not necessary when "one purpose of the testing is to evaluate decisional capacity." Further, the Ethics Code states:

> For persons who are legally incapable of giving informed consent, psychologists nevertheless (1) provide an appropriate explanation, (2) seek the individual's assent, (3) consider such persons' preferences and best interests, and (4) obtain appropriate permission from a legally authorized person, if such substitute consent is permitted or required by law. When consent by a legally authorized person is not permitted or required by law, psychologists take reasonable steps to protect the individual's rights and welfare.

Part of the consent process also includes discussion of who will be privy to test results (e.g., if testing is requested by an interdisciplinary team, or through the court), and that the older adult's confidentiality will be respected to the extent possible in the current situation. In interdisciplinary care settings (e.g., rehabilitation unit, nursing home), older patients should be aware that the team will be privy to test results as appropriate.

Other ethical issues relevant to geropsychological assessment include close attention to the reliability and validity of test results. Many commonly used psychological tests have not been appropriately normed with older populations and should be used cautiously with older adults. Similarly, older adults with limited educational backgrounds, whose first language is not English, or who are from different cultural backgrounds may not be fairly evaluated by commonly used standardized tests (Manly, 2006; Manly, Byrd, Touradji, & Stern, 2004). For example, depressive symptoms may present differently in older adults from different ethnic/racial backgrounds (Ganguli & Hendrie, 2005; Skarupski et al., 2005). Geropsychologists take great care to appreciate the potential impact of sensory or motor deficits and environmental distractions on test performance.

In addition, ethical geropsychology assessment and intervention practice entail appropriate coding and billing for services provided, which often entails billing Medicare (for further discussion, see Vacha-Haase's chapter, "Teaching, Supervision, and the Business of Geropsychology" in this volume). The APA Practice Directorate Web site (www.apapractice. org) is a good resource for information on working with Medicare, as is the Center for Medicare and Medicaid Services Web site (www.cms.org; Hartman-Stein & Georgoulakis, 2007).

INTERVENTION

Ethical considerations for psychological intervention include informed consent, confidentiality, privacy, and advocacy.

Just as in the case of geropsychological assessment, geropsychologists obtain informed consent from older adults (or their legal surrogates) for psychotherapy or other psychological treatments (e.g., behavioral or environmental interventions). The APA Ethics Code provisions for informed consent for psychotherapy apply to psychotherapy with older adults. These standards include that "psychologists inform clients/patients as early as is feasible in the therapeutic relationship about the nature and anticipated course of therapy, fees, involvement of third parties, and limits of confidentiality and provide sufficient opportunity for the client/patient to ask questions and receive answers" (American Psychological Association, 2002b, pp. 14–15). In addition, geropsychology trainees inform older adult clients that they are working under supervision. In some care settings, older adults may not be seeking psychological services for themselves but rather are referred by health care teams or family members. In these cases, it is equally if not more important for the older adult (or legal surrogate) to understand who the psychologist is, the condition being addressed, what services are being offered, and the possible consequences of accepting or refusing services. The older adult must then have the opportunity to consent, assent, or decline services (Coverdale, McCullough, Molinari, & Workman, 2006; Lichtenberg et al., 1998).

The ethical standard of confidentiality can pose many challenges in geriatric mental health care. Older adults have the same right to confidentiality of psychological services as adults of any age. However, with greater likelihood of either family involvement or interdisciplinary team care in working with older adults, negotiating issues of confidentiality can be challenging (Karel, 2008; Lichtenberg et al., 1998; Norris, 2002). During informed consent, older adults must be informed of the limits of confidentiality. Confidentiality exceptions include those made for safety concerns, legal requirements for reporting elder and child abuse, and HIPAA (Health Insurance Portability and Accountability Act, see www.apapractice.org/apo/hipaa.html#), Medicare, or other insurer regulations regarding medical record documentation.

Further, older adults treated in inpatient medical, rehabilitation, long-term care, or residential settings must be informed about interdisciplinary treatment planning and requirements for documentation that will be shared with the team. It can help to discuss with the older adult that sharing some information with the team may lead to improved care overall. Psychologists often assist older adults by helping other members of the health care team to respond most appropriately to the elder's particular values, goals, capacities, fears, and preferred styles of coping. On the other hand, it is important to collaborate with the older adult in defining what information is appropriate, or not, to share with the treatment team. In general, a good rule of thumb is to document information as generally as possible and adopt a "need to know" principle—communicate only information that is essential to the patient's care (Norris, 2002).

Likewise, it can be difficult to negotiate communication with family members. Concerned family members may assume that you will talk with them about the older adult's care, and they often need to be educated that it is the older adult's decision about how much, if any, information is shared (if the older adult has the capacity to make that decision). Some older adults are very comfortable with and want their family members to be part of their mental health care; others wish to maintain clear boundaries. In many cases, including family members in the mental health treatment can be very helpful, especially if there are concerns about the older adult's self-care, and couples and family interventions are often indicated. It is tricky when an older adult refuses to have family members involved, particularly when it is clear that intervening at the family system level would be most productive. Ultimately, a decisionally intact older adult has the right to make this decision. It is important, at the beginning of psychological treatment, to clarify with the older adult who it is permissible to communicate with under particular circumstances. For example, older adults with hearing impairments often prefer to have a family member help with scheduling appointments over the phone, even if they do not wish the family member to participate in therapy.

Older adults have a right to privacy in delivery of psychological services (American Psychological Association, 2002b; Lichtenberg et al., 1998). In some care settings, however, private spaces can be difficult to find. Particularly in hospital, nursing home, or other inpatient settings, patients often have roommates and, if patients are able to get out of bed, it can be difficult to find private office space. In general, it is important to coordinate as much as possible with nursing staff (e.g., to help a resident out of bed if appropriate), roommates (if possible, a roommate can be asked to leave the room for a period of time), and other users of space (can an office be borrowed for a particular period of time). The older adult ultimately can decide if and where she is comfortable to meet given possible constraints on privacy.

Finally, geropsychologists often play an important advocacy role— within systems and for individual patients—to help ensure appropriate delivery of health, mental health, and social services for older adults. The *Standards for Psychological Services in Long-Term Care Facilities* (Lichtenberg et al., 1998) emphasizes the importance of psychologists serving as advocates for provision of clinically appropriate mental health services for older adults in long-term care settings. Appropriate services are based on clinical necessity, on a biopsychosocial framework for assessment and treatment, and are consistent with the most current research and clinical guidelines (Karel, 2008). As health and social service care systems can be very difficult to access and negotiate, psychologists act as advocates for their older clients' access to needed services (e.g., by providing information, referral, care coordination, education, and communication with other care providers) but are careful to encourage older adults to act as advocates for themselves as much as they are able.

CONSULTATION

Geropsychologists frequently serve as consultants to families, primary care providers, health care teams, long-term care facilities, social service agencies, and agencies dedicated to local and national health care and social service policy for older adults. Given that older adults often have complex and interacting challenges (e.g., chronic medical illness, physical disability, mental illness, dementia, social service needs), they often require integrated care by a team of professionals. The American Psychological Association recently published a report, *Blueprint for Change: Achieving Integrated Health Care for an Aging Population* (American Psychological Association Presidential Task Force on Integrated Health Care for an Aging Population, 2008), that reviewed the important role psychologists can play in providing integrated care. Part of this role entails providing consultation, education, and training in multidisciplinary team settings.

Consultation to teams or organizations can raise specific ethical dilemmas, as addressed by the APA Ethics Code (2002b) and the Pikes Peak Model competencies. Consultants often must recognize and negotiate multiple roles, and potential conflicts of interest. Per the APA Ethics Code, Standard 3.11 addresses the issue of psychological services delivered to or through organizations, as follows:

> (a) Psychologists delivering services to or through organizations provide information beforehand to clients and when appropriate those directly affected by the services about (1) the nature and objectives of the services, (2) the intended recipients, (3) which of the individuals are clients, (4) the relationship the psychologist will have with each person and the organization, (5) the probable uses of services provided and information obtained, (6) who will have access to the information, and (7) limits of confidentiality. As soon as feasible, they provide information about the results and conclusions of such services to appropriate persons.
>
> (b) If psychologists will be precluded by law or by organizational roles from providing such information to particular individuals or groups, they so inform those individuals or groups at the outset of the service.

These guidelines are applicable to geropsychology consultation practice. Similar clarifications are often necessary when geropsychologists are consulting with the family of an older adult (e.g., making recommendations about how best to manage dementia-related behaviors). In long-term care settings, there are often conflicting goals in terms of the interests of the facility versus the interests of the resident. Psychologists consulting to long-term care settings frequently encounter the tension between promoting the older adult's autonomy (often the primary value and goal of the patient) and protecting her safety (often the primary value and goal of the institution; Karel, 2008). The *Standards for Psychological Services in Long-Term Care Facilities* (Lichtenberg et al., 1998) states: "Psychologists are aware that at times the interests of the facility and the patient may not coincide and make every effort to resolve the conflict in the best interests of the patient" (p. 126).

Conflicts of interest also arise when necessary services are not reimbursed by third-party payers. In particular, optimal mental health care in interdisciplinary care settings typically requires some time to meet with the team (to obtain necessary clinical information, share psychological conceptualizations and recommendations, coordinate care). Time for team meetings is not reimbursed. Again, according to Psychologists in Long Term Care (PLTC) standards, geropsychologists resolve these conflicts in the best interest of the patient and advocate for policy changes that will lead to optimal care for long-term care residents.

RESEARCH

Geropsychologists are aware of ethical issues regarding research with potentially vulnerable older adults. Ongoing research is critical to help advance knowledge about geriatric health, mental health, and assessment and treatment, including knowledge about disabling conditions such as dementia and severe mental illness in late life. However, individuals with these conditions may not have the capacity to provide informed consent to participate in research studies. The research community is working to find a balance between pursuing important research and providing human subject protections for vulnerable elders. Several efforts have been made to provide recommendations to researchers and Institutional Review Boards (Alzheimer's Association, 2004; Kim et al., 2004). For example, these recommendations address when to include cognitively impaired individuals in research, strategies for evaluating capacity for research consent, and the role of surrogates in providing proxy consent for research participation.

Recent research examined the attitudes of patients with Alzheimer's disease and their study partners regarding proxy consent for a clinical medication trial (Karlawish et al., 2008b). The majority of participants, both patients and partners, supported the notion of proxy consent for study participation. Study partners reported that they made decisions about participation based on what they thought was best for the patient rather than using a substituted judgment standard (i.e., trying to imagine what the patient would have wanted). In the same research program, a structured capacity assessment interview was helpful in determining the capacity of patients with Alzheimer's disease to consent to the clinical trial (Karlawish et al., 2008a).

A Model for Negotiating Ethical Dilemmas

The Pikes Peak foundational ethical competency recommends that geropsychologists "understand and apply ethical and legal standards," referring to the range of ethical issues discussed in this chapter. In considering how to "apply" ethical and legal standards, geropsychologists may turn to many models of ethical decision making. Here, I provide a simple framework that integrates the core features of many decision-making models (Cassel, Mezey, & Bottrell, 2002; Doolittle & Herrick, 1992; Fox, Berkowitz, Chanko, & Powell, 2005; Hanson, Kerkoff, & Bush, 2005; Holstein & Mitzen, 2001; Jonsen, Siegler, & Winslade, 1998; Karel & Moye, 2006) and takes into account that identification and resolution of ethical dilemmas in geriatric care often occur in the context of multiple stakeholders: older adult patient, family members, health care team with varying perspectives, agency rules and regulations, as well as the psychologist's own professional and personal values.

Psychologists apply ethical and legal standards in their work all the time, often without thinking explicitly about it. It is when there are ethical dilemmas, or conflicting notions about what is the right thing to do in a specific situation, that we become particularly mindful of our ethics code, local policies, and laws, and look for a systematic way of clarifying and

---

Approximately 1 year after his return home after rehabilitation for his fractured leg, Mr. Sanders was not doing as well. His son continued to help weekly with his bills and medications but was becoming more concerned about his dad's repetitive questions, anxious mood, and increasingly poor housekeeping. He felt he didn't have the time to address his father's increasing needs for assistance. His daughter thought he sounded okay during their daily phone calls, but, during her recent visit, she was surprised to see a messy house, her father's weight loss, and the absence of his usual spark. He spent much of his time sitting and watching television, which was not typical for her active father. She went out for a drive with her father, and was startled to note his erratic driving behavior.

Mr. Sanders' son and daughter arranged for a visit to his primary care doctor, who was concerned about possible depression and/or dementia and referred Mr. Sanders to a geriatric mental health clinic affiliated with the medical center. He met several times with the clinic geropsychologist (and, with his permission, his son joined one meeting) and consulted with the geropsychiatrist. They concluded that Mr. Sanders likely had early dementia as well as mixed anxiety/depression and recommended psychotherapy, a neurology consult, and a family meeting to discuss Mr. Sanders' living situation and needs for support at this time. At the meeting, which Mr. Sanders' daughter joined by conference

> *call, the geropsychologist realized it was going to be difficult to reach consensus regarding planning for the future. She provided feedback about initial diagnostic impressions and expressed concern about Mr. Sanders' degree of independent living and driving. Mr. Sanders admitted some concern but promised he would try harder, that he really wanted to stay home and drive and not bother his children. While Mr. Sanders' daughter felt they should look into assisted living options, or a move in with her or her brother, and have her father stop driving, his son was very torn about taking away his father's independence. Mr. Sanders' primary care provider had clearly recommended that Mr. Sanders stop driving and investigate a more supervised living situation at this time.*

intervening in ethically or legally ambiguous situations. To illustrate a simple ethical decision-making framework here, let's return to the case of Mr. Sanders, introduced earlier in the chapter.

An ethical decision-making framework applied to this clinical situation might look like this (Karel, 2008b):

Step 1. Clarify the ethical issue. What is the dilemma? Who is concerned, and who thinks which aspects of the situation are problematic? What clinical information is important and relevant to the issue at hand? "Often it can be very helpful simply to define the problem; sometimes clarifying the problem, and the differing perspectives, in a clear, compassionate, and respectful way can help all parties involved realize that they share a number of concerns" (Karel, 2008b, p. 118).

> *In this case, it is important to clarify that everyone involved is interested in Mr. Sanders' health, well-being, and quality of life, as well as his safety and the safety of others. The dilemma is how best to address all of these values and goals. Clinically important information is that Mr. Sanders has shown a significant decline in his cognitive and functional abilities over the past year or so, likely attributable to a progressive dementia and perhaps exacerbated by depression and anxiety. Information about his other medical problems, coping resources, social supports, and functioning at home and in the community is all important and relevant.*

Step 2. Clarify who are the relevant stakeholders and each of their values, goals, and interests. A systematic review of who is genuinely concerned and affected by particular outcomes is important to guide ethical decision making. This review can include consideration of patient and family preferences regarding quality of life and contextual concerns; health care team concerns and preferences related to individual providers' personal and professional values, as well as concerns about professional responsibility and liability; and legitimate community-based concerns about safety (e.g., unsafe drivers or apartment dwellers who may put other tenants at risk).

> *Mr. Sanders is obviously the primary stakeholder in decisions about his living situation and ability to drive, and the impact of these issues on his independence, privacy, financial situation, and quality of life. His children are also legitimate stakeholders, in that different options for his care (e.g., moving in with one of them, increased help at home, move to assisted living) may have a significant impact on their time, money, family relationships, and relationships with their father. Additionally, Mr. Sanders' health care providers, including the psychologist, have a legitimate interest in his well-being given their professional responsibilities, and they also bring specific values and preferences to such situations. Finally, the community has a stake in the safety of drivers on the road.*

Step 3. Clarify decision-making authority. Who has the right to make the decision in a particular situation? Sometimes stakeholders may disagree, yet it remains clear whose decision it is to make. An individual with intact decision-making capacity has the right to make decisions about his own affairs as long as he does not pose undue burden on or risk to others. Sometimes, when a capable patient makes an unpopular decision, an open discussion can help explore why others are concerned, and clarify different options. If a patient is marginally capable, this step should include efforts to optimize that person's participation in decision making, through eliciting his values, fears, goals, and preferences (Carpenter et al., 2007; Karel, Moye, et al., 2007). If a patient is clearly not capable of making decisions for himself, then a surrogate decision maker must be identified. In complex cases, health care teams may have concerns over a surrogate's capacity to make decisions, and/or a surrogate's motivation to act in the best interest of a patient. In these cases, it is often helpful to involve institutional ethics committees.

An important question in Mr. Sanders's case is whether he maintains the capacities to (1) live safely alone and drive and (2) to make decisions about living and driving, based on his ability to understand and appreciate his abilities. Rarely are these clear "black and white" situations. Mr. Sanders' health care team lets him know that he needs more help to live alone, and that he (after further evaluation) should not be driving. Let's say that he refuses to believe this assessment and insists that everyone should leave him alone and let him be. In such a case, further evaluation might demonstrate that he does not currently have the capacity to understand, appreciate, and reason through the risks and benefits of options regarding residential and driving decisions. At his last hospital stay, he had designated his son to be his health care proxy, but he does not have a legal guardian who would have the power to make a range of life decisions on his behalf. If Mr. Sanders, with the help of his children and his health care team, was not able or willing to be part of a process of reaching consensus, then perhaps legal mechanisms might be used to grant another the power to make decisions on his behalf.

Step 4. Consider all ethically justifiable options. What are the pros and cons of each option in meeting the values and goals of the stakeholders? Often, this process of open communication and demonstration of respect for the concerns of all involved can lead to a plan of action that is acceptable to everyone.

An elder services social worker helped Mr. Sanders and his family to understand the wide range of options to help him be safe while optimizing his quality of life. Options included bringing more services into Mr. Sanders' home (e.g., meals-on-wheels, homemaking assistance, volunteer companion), making use of adult day programs, considering a move to the daughter's (not ideal as she lived in a part of the country unfamiliar to him) or son's (possible, but challenging given the son's family and space issues in his small house), exploring assisted living options in the community (he would have to sell his home to help fund this option), and having another formal driving evaluation to determine driving safety at this time. Although Mr. Sanders had trouble appreciating the extent of the family's and psychologist's concerns for him, he was able to clearly express that he values staying in his own home as long as possible and living near his friends and church. He repeatedly expressed his concern about being a burden to his children. All agreed that after he was treated for depression and anxiety, he might be better able to consider his options. For the short term, everyone agreed that he would receive increased services in his home and a moratorium on driving until the formal evaluation. Mr. Sanders also agreed that he would be willing to try an adult day program to get out of the house and more actively involved with others his age. Mr. Sanders also agreed that he would like to give his son power of attorney to manage his financial interests. His daughter agreed that she would start investigating assisted living options should the plan for him to stay at home not work now or in the future.

Step 5: Implement, evaluate, and reevaluate. It is important to follow up and evaluate whether the plan chosen has addressed the concerns of the patient, family, and other stakeholders. In the case of ethical dilemmas for older adults with dementia, the individual's capacities and needs for care continue to change, and thus the appropriate solutions continue to change as well. Therefore, decisions often need to be reevaluated over time and adjusted for changes in an individual's decision-making abilities and needs for assistance.

For several months, Mr. Sanders was able to function safely at home. He unhappily stopped driving, but was able to use the town's senior van to get to and from the day program as well as to his medical appointments in town. Over time, however, he had increasing difficulty managing his self-care and his family needed to pursue options for assisted living and, later, skilled nursing care.

Conclusions

Ethical geropsychology practice requires knowledge and skill competencies that may be relatively unfamiliar to psychologists who do not work often with older adults and care systems. This chapter has reviewed some of the distinctive ethical and legal issues that arise, especially in the care of vulnerable older adults, particularly those with cognitive or psychiatric disabilities that compromise decision-making capacity. Psychologists working with older adults must be familiar with the concept and assessment of decision-making capacity, the mechanisms and challenges of surrogate decision making, and the clinical, legal, and social tools available to help promote dignity and protect the safety of vulnerable elders.

Assessment, intervention, consultation, and research with older adult populations, as well as families and related care systems, all demand special ethical considerations. Issues including informed consent, confidentiality, privacy, conflicts of interest, and appropriate billing and documentation are all important. At times, these basic ethical principles can be difficult to safeguard in working with complex older adults and care systems. A five-step model to guide the process of ethical decision making in working with older adults was provided. Additionally, throughout the chapter, many resources including useful Web sites were referenced that provide practical information and guidance for psychologists working to enhance their competence for ethical geropsychology practice.

TEN

Teaching, Supervision, and the Business of Geropsychology

Tammi Vacha-Haase

Following his attendance at the 2005 White House Conference on Aging representing the American Psychological Association (APA) as its president, Levant (2008) highlighted several of the implementation strategies discussed that had the potential to directly impact the future of education in psychology. The most salient included national resolutions to "Attain adequate numbers of health care personnel in all professions who are skilled, culturally competent and specialized in geriatrics" and to "Support geriatric education and training for all health care professionals, paraprofessionals, health professional students and direct care workers" (Levant, 2008, p. 95).

Transformation can already be seen in the present marketplace, and current day advertisements demonstrate the enormous attention given to the multiple training and employment opportunities, including research, clinical practice, teaching, and services targeted at the elderly. Although working with the aging is not always viewed as a "glamorous" area of study, the past few decades have brought about a dramatic increase of offerings in the area of aging, addressing the later stages of the life span in both undergraduate and graduate courses. With these increasing educational opportunities, the need is ever present for competent geropsychologists with a commitment to teaching and supervision. These individuals must be skilled in providing appropriate training for those interested in learning about older adults, whether on an applied or professional level, at a place of business or an academic institution. The training that these geropsychologists offer must be based on a clear assessment of their learning needs in regard to stage of training, amount of experience, and/or discipline. Whether at an undergraduate, graduate, or post-graduate level, today's geropsychologists are actively engaged in the teaching, supervision, clinical, and business aspects of the profession.

Teaching: Undergraduate Education

The field of adult development and aging has countless applications throughout the field of psychology. Many universities now offer certificates or degrees specializing in adult development and aging, in addition to specialized courses across the life span, both in the classroom as well as online (Mehrotra & Fried, 2002).

Following a traditional model, Hulicka and Whitbourne (1990) identified five major goals for an introductory course in adult development and aging, suggesting that a course of this type include the following:

1. A multidisciplinary perspective of the psychological, social, and biological aspects of aging
2. Scientific investigation in gerontology
3. Self-awareness
4. Opportunities to gain experiences interacting with aging adults outside of the classroom
5. Application of class information to future career possibilities

Those teaching an undergraduate course in aging are encouraged to refer to the homepage of the Division of Adult Development of Aging (Division 20) of APA at http://apadiv20.phhp.ufl.edu/#. This site provides a wealth of support materials for educators, including teaching tips, an updated (although not reviewed) list of textbooks, educational videos, and examples of submitted syllabi.

A recent review (January 2009) of these undergraduate syllabi provided on the division's Web site (http://apadiv20.phhp.ufl.edu/syllugrd.htm) indicated overlap with the themes suggested by Hulicka and Whitbourne (1990) in the course goals for adult development and aging. The majority of courses identified the purpose of the class as increasing knowledge within a theoretical framework of later life development, with a caveat that the class would go beyond theory to applied knowledge. The majority of syllabi indicated that the course explored the biological, psychological, and social factors associated with aging and the aged. Topics tended to include theories of aging, normative and non-normative biological changes, cognitive functioning, personality, psycho-social issues, meaning in late life, death, and dying. The instructors of these courses also tended to highlight the importance of thinking critically about issues pertaining to aging, as the majority of course syllabi included topics on research, clinical, and policy issues. Many instructors appeared to have students utilize existing literature through an evaluative lens "to develop a critical appreciation for the existing psychological research." Another general goal identified by reviewing the selected syllabi included the importance of students examining their personal attitudes regarding older persons.

Of further note was the trend to include a course goal of recognizing individual differences among older persons as well as understanding how culture and time period shape the experience of adulthood. Today's changing demographics in American society would suggest that the majority of students will find themselves working with an older population that is larger in numbers, older in age, and more diverse than ever before; thus, class topics on the uniqueness of the individual and cultural context would seem appropriate.

A somewhat newer addition to several syllabi appeared to be the promotion of positive views on aging, with an additional spotlight on advancing optimal functioning. Instructors of these courses tended to focus on successful aging, accenting their conviction that older age should not be synonymous with decline, frailty, and death. Given that the older population is living longer and healthier than ever before, students' recognition of the healthy aspects of aging will be vital in their work with older adults.

Consensus in the choice of textbook for teaching an undergraduate aging course appears challenging. Although a number of options are available, Ferraro (2006) listed the five most recommended textbooks for an undergraduate course. These included Cavanaugh and Blanchard-Fields (2006), Erber (2005), Foos and Clark (2003), Lemme (2006), and Hoyer and Roodin (2003).

As previously noted, the psychology of adult development and aging is often taught at the undergraduate level as a specialized course. However, progressive instruction suggests that aging be included in all psychology courses, from introduction of general psychology, to research methods, to social psychology, to cognitive and neurosciences. Whitbourne and Cavanaugh (2003) edited a book providing practical instruction for integrating aging and adult development content into psychology courses. The authors focused on aging topics both in the core curriculum, such as abnormal psychology, and in more specialized areas, such as gender and industrial/organizational psychology.

This comprehensive approach to undergraduate teaching provides broader coverage, as well as a more accurate reflection of society and the area of psychology. The increasing aging population, and thereby potential for students to interact with older adults regardless of their future career goals, provides additional relevance for inclusion in all psychology courses. For example, a course on the psychology of human sexuality should include information about the sexual response of older adults. Although changes in physical appearance and sensory acuity may feed the stereotype of the elderly as asexual, research indicates that intimacy and sexuality are an important part of healthy relationships throughout the life span. A basic human sexuality course will no doubt be improved by covering the age-related physiological change in the sex response cycle, as well as including information challenging stereotypes, such as, contrary to popular belief, these changes do not signal the end of a satisfying sex life, and many older adults enjoy intimacy and physical contact throughout their lives. A course on sensation and perception could be enhanced by including information regarding the sensory process of older adults and changes during the later stages of life. Utilizing examples of research from the aging literature, or including older adults when providing illustrative examples, will give research methods and statistic courses a far-reaching appeal. More clinically focused undergraduate courses, such as introduction to helping skills or professional issues in addictive treatment, will be a richer learning experience with class material that includes older adults.

Training Psychologists to Work With Older Adults

Almost three decades ago, Santos and VandenBos (1982) recognized the importance of training doctoral-level psychologists to work with the elderly. Since then, many (e.g., Fretz, 1993; Hinrichsen, Myers, & Stewart, 2000; Jacobs & Formati, 1998; Qualls, 1998) have affirmed this call to action, highlighting the need to train psychologists competent to work with an aging adult population. Early predictions projected that approximately 7,500 full-time psychologists would be necessary to meet the growing demands of this aging population (Gatz & Finkel, 1995). Taking a slightly more conservative approach, APA estimated a need for 5,000 psychologists with this specialty by 2020. However, a clear gap was identified in 2002 as practice patterns among APA members revealed that only 3% of licensed psychologists worked primarily with older adults, although 69% had older adults among their clientele (Qualls, Segal, Norman, Niederehe, &

Gallagher-Thompson, 2002). Unfortunately, even as this chapter is being written, little has appeared to change, as only a limited number of practicing psychologists identify as specializing with older adults (National Register of Health Service Providers in Psychology, 2009).

It should be remembered, however, that psychologists do not have to specialize in geropsychology to work with older clients (Knight, Karel, Hinrichsen, Qualls, & Duffy, 2009). Let's assume that the average full-time clinician at any given time has a caseload of 50 patients (not all are seen weekly), and that by 2030, one out of five people in this nation will be 65 years of age. Basic math suggests that the average practitioner would then have a caseload including approximately 10 patients who are age 65 or older. These calculations suggest that it is not unreasonable to estimate that at a minimum, a general practitioner in the future would spend one full day a week providing services to older adults.

But what do these practitioners need to know to be competent to treat older adults? Perhaps Qualls (1998) provided a beginning response to this question: "The answer depends on the level of specialty services one needs to provide" (p. 24). Which begs a number of additional questions: What are the services that psychologists with a general practice provide for older adults? How do these services differ from those that geropsychologists provide? What is the best approach to training these clinicians? What can be done to increase the number of psychologists who are competent to work with older adults?

Unfortunately, there are no easy answers. But what is clear is that whether it is during their graduate education, their internship, or after they have completed their degree, competent psychologists in the future will need to possess a knowledge base and skill set to provide a variety of services across different settings to an older adult population.

PREDOCTORAL EDUCATION

In the early 1980s Lubin and his colleagues (Lubin, Brady, Thomas, & Whitlock, 1986) surveyed APA-accredited clinical, counseling, and combined doctoral programs to explore the availability of geropsychology training compared to the findings of a study completed a decade earlier (Siegler, Gentry, & Edwards, 1979). Results indicated a modest and consistent increase in course and practica offerings; and perhaps most promising, 11 programs, rather than just one in 1975, offered a subspecialty in geropsychology. A decade later, this trend continued, as approximately 20 APA-accredited clinical and counseling psychology programs (out of about 250) offered specialized training in aging (Blieszner, 1994).

Regardless of the consistent, albeit slow, growth in the number of graduate programs offering geropsychology training in these earlier studies, today advancement in academic training now appears to have stalled. In an attempt to identify programs with clinical geropsychology training opportunities, researchers made calls in the summer of 2003 to a number of listservs requesting information identifying those graduate programs providing educational opportunities in geropsychology. In the end, the final list included only 11 formal programs (e.g., those with a primary geropsychology focus, "track," "emphasis," "proficiency, " "concentration," "area of interest," or "minor" in geropsychology) and two informal programs (those that offer opportunities to work with geropsychologists within an applied psychology graduate program or with geropsychologists in other programs). A listing of these programs can be found at geropsych. org/Student%20Graduate%20Education%20Page.htm.

Although some (e.g., Hinrichsen & Zweig, 2005) remain optimistic about the gradual growth in opportunities in geropsychology education and training within psychology doctoral programs, the relatively low number of programs included in the above list remains a concern, and something of a mystery given that students respond well to such offerings. Karel and her colleagues (Karel, Molinari, Gallagher-Thompson, & Hillman, 1999) found that 47% of those psychologists who pursued specialty-level training in clinical geropsychology began their interest during graduate school. Significant influences on students' interest in the field included work experience (65%), research experience (49%), and coursework (32%). Others (Koder & Helmes, 2008) identified clinical exposure to older adult clients and age-related course content as influencing factors for Australian psychologists who specialized with older adults. Hinrichsen and McMeniman (2002) noted that when compared to trainees without a geropsychology placement, those trainees provided a geropsychology practicum experience maintained a higher interest in geropsychology, as well as lower negative attitudes toward older people, perhaps decreasing what Duffy and Morales (1997) referred to as trainee "gerophobia." In sum, research supports the conclusion that professional geropsychology would benefit if graduate programs integrated aging issues into current courses (e.g., psychopathology or research design), added a course in adult development and aging, and/or offered geropsychology practicum opportunities (Hinrichsen, 2000).

As early as 1984 Lewinsohn and his colleagues (Lewinsohn, Teri, & Hautzinger, 1984) shared their experiences of creating a "geropsychological services program" in hopes that this would provide others with the needed information, or at least a beginning structure, to implement this type of training. Over the years, numerous others (e.g., Duffy, 1992; Qualls, Duffy, & Crose, 1995; Vacha-Haase & Duffy, in press) have described a practicum model that is designed to provide intensive geropsychology experience to doctoral students. Program examples have been published, from how to maintain a general focus while infusing aging training (DeVries, 2005), to how to build a specialist geropsychology doctoral program (Qualls, Segal, Benight, & Kenny, 2005).

INTERNSHIP AND POSTDOCTORAL TRAINING

In addition to graduate education in the area of geropsychology, experience can be obtained both at the internship and postdoctoral levels. The Association of Psychology Postdoctoral and Internship Centers (APPIC) organization oversees the National Match Program for predoctoral internship sites and also provides information on postdoctoral opportunities. The 2008–09 Directory (retrieved from www.appic.org/downloads/ APPIC_Directory_08_09.pdf), as well as those in future years, are available for download through the Web site (www.appic.org/about/2_2_about_ organizational_information.html). Interested trainees can explore these listings to locate the most up-to-date information regarding internship sites with major rotations in geropsychology or older adults. A search of the Web site (APPIC, 2008) offered options to find internship sites for "older adults" as the specified type of client population, or by "geropsychology" as a specialty area. As of January 2009, 161 internship sites offered major rotations working with older adults; 444 offered minor rotations with this population. When specifying "geropsychology" as the specialty area, 113 sites offered major rotations and 309 sites offered minor rotations.

Although fairly limited at the current time, postdoctoral-level geropsychology training opportunities do exist for those seeking this type of educational experience. A search of the Web site (APPIC, 2008) in January of 2009 identified 74 postdoctoral sites available for working with "older adults," and 45 postdoctoral sites were listed as having "geropsychology" as a specialty area.

Viable opportunities for geropsychology postdoctoral training occur across a range of medical and psychiatric settings, with the most frequently reported primary training settings including outpatient geriatric mental health clinics (74% reported some training in that setting), nursing homes (64%), neuropsychology services (62%), geriatric multidisciplinary outpatient evaluation settings (46%), inpatient geropsychiatry units (45%), and geriatric inpatient medical evaluation settings (45%; Karel et al., 1999).

Internship and postdoctoral training in geropsychology can also be offered through multisite, multilevel programs (Hyer, Leventhal, & Gartenberg, 2005) and nursing home settings (Karel & Moye, 2005). The Department of Veterans Administration (DVA) offers a number of geropsychology experiences, and many geropsychologists have completed internship and postdoctoral programs through the DVA system (Karel et al., 1999).

Offering rotations or adding geropsychology to current training has been recommended as a highly valuable option to current training sites. In a presentation to APPIC, Karel (2007b) encouraged internship sites to provide geropsychology training "To develop interest, skills, and knowledge of geropsychology . . . to provide opportunities for experiential application of knowledge; to promote professional development and identity of the trainee as a geropsychologist; to prepare the intern for future career development. Upon exiting the internship, the trainee will not be expected to be an expert in all areas of geropsychology but should be competent in the areas in which they received training" (Karel, 2007b, slide 20). She provided recommendations for the initial competency assessment of interns, clinical settings, didactics, and faculty resources. Karel (2007b) also called for postdoctoral training sites to meet the needs of psychologists at two levels. The first "for those who come in with incrementally obtained and substantive preparation, to reach a level of advanced practice in geropsychology and/or entry into research, academic, or training roles" and another "for those with lesser degrees of geropsychology preparation/exposure, to transition to full autonomous professional functioning and competence in geropsychology practice or research" (Karel, 2007b, slide 22).

Rather than completing internships and postdoctoral training, some practicing psychologists may find that by necessity they have slowly become "the geropsychologist" for their group practice or place of employment. Others, at some point in their career may decide to expand their practice to include older adults, or even choose to develop a specialty in working with an older population. Experienced therapists may be more likely to complete further education to gain additional skills in working with older adults if they are reminded of the importance of the body of knowledge of general clinical training, recognizing basic human emotions and dynamics that can transcend across age, gender, or ethnicity (Duffy & Morales, 1997). Duffy (1992) warned against the tendency to underestimate the generalizability of one's clinical skills and competency to help patients, regardless of age. Thus, those interested in adding specific geropsychology skills to their general clinical competence can accomplish this by finding training in working with older adults through APA, and more recently through private companies, as continuing education credits are often offered at local or regional workshops, as pre-convention offerings, and even through distance learning. The Clinical Geropsychology, Division 12, Section II Web site (http://geropsych.org/students.t.html) provides listings of continuing education offered through the Continuing Education Committee of APA's Division 20 and Division 12, and Psychologists in Long Term Care (PLTC).

TRAINING RESOURCES

A number of resources have been developed to assist with the training of professional psychologists working with older adults. The Guidelines for Psychological Practice with Older Adults (APA, 2004) were intended to build on the APA's Ethical Principles of Psychologists and Code of Conduct and other APA policies. These guidelines were authored to aid psychologists in providing services to older adults, by offering practitioners "(a) a frame of reference for engaging in clinical work with older adults and (b) basic information and further references in the areas of attitudes, general aspects of aging, clinical issues, assessment, intervention, consultation, and continuing education and training relative to work with older adults" (APA, 2004, p. 237).

Building on these guidelines, the Pikes Peak Model (Knight et al., 2009) is the most recent contribution in the area of training in professional geropsychology and provides a training model for educating competent geropsychologists to provide services to an aging population. An aspirational, competencies-based approach in training to work with older adults, this model allows for entry points at multiple levels of professional development, acknowledging that entry into geropsychology training can occur at various stages of a psychologist's career and that there are many pathways in which to achieve competency. The spirit of the model centers on inclusivity, with an "open door" for generalist practitioners to enhance their competence working with aging clients. Focus is given to professional geropsychology competencies, consisting of attitudes, knowledge, and skills for working with older adults. Six key elements for training in professional geropsychology were outlined:

1. Trainees are taught about the normal aging process

2. Bona fide professional "geropsychologists" are utilized for direct supervision

3. Trainees are provided diverse experiences to increase self-awareness in the area of human differences

4. Trainees are exposed to the variety of settings where older adults are treated (e.g., hospitals, long-term care facilities, client home)

5. Focus is given to the interdisciplinary and team approach to treatment necessary when working with older adults

6. Ethical and legal issues unique to geropsychology are highlighted

As detailed in Molinari's chapter, Professional Identification", in this volume, the Pikes Peak conference also served as the catalyst for the establishment of the Council of Professional Geropsychology Training Programs (CoPGTP; http://www.usc.edu/programs/cpgtp/). Now with over 30 members, CoPGTP includes programs and individuals that provide geropsychology training in psychology graduate, internship, and postdoctoral programs as well training to post-licensure psychologists. CoPGTP is committed to the promotion of excellence in and the development of high-quality training programs in professional geropsychology. CoPGTP is especially interested in facilitating access to resources in the acquisition of geropsychology knowledge and skill competencies among licensed psychologists who want to acquire them later in their careers.

Highlighted Areas of Supervision in Professional Geropsychology

The Pike's Peak Model noted that not all psychologists who treat older adult clients require specific training in geropsychology. In fact, many clinicians will work as effectively with older clients as younger clients presenting with similar clinical issues. However, more complex clinical cases with some older clients will require an in-depth understanding of life-span changes, late-life psychopathologies, chronic medical conditions, and age-driven social and environmental contexts.

TEACHING AND SUPERVISING CLINICAL SKILLS

As noted previously, working with an older adult population does not require an entire new set of clinical or professional skills (Duffy & Morales, 1997). However, supervisors must be attentive to many unique clinical skills included in geropsychology.

Rapport Competency

First, a competent geropsychologist must be able to relate effectively and empathically with older adults and their families. Additional expertise to form effective working alliances with a wide range of older clients, families, colleagues, and other stakeholders is required in establishing a therapeutic relationship. In his seminal book *Psychotherapy with Older Adults*, Knight (2004) dedicated an entire chapter to establishing rapport with older clients. He highlighted the need for understanding older clients within their contextual cohort and integrating this with an educational approach about psychotherapy. That is, the competent geropsychologist remains aware of the historical influences affecting particular cohorts, as the understanding of the broad historical timeline of events that may have influenced an elderly person's perspective on life is paramount. A general awareness of the social impact of wars, the Great Depression, and other historical events may help clients to feel that the therapist is interested in understanding their stage in life. When working to form a therapeutic alliance with an older client, a competent geropsychologist should take into account the unique experience of each person based on demographic, sociocultural, and life experiences, and understand that multiple factors interact over the life span to influence an older individual's patterns of behavior.

Those working with older clients must also recognize that older adults often face multiple challenges in obtaining counseling services due to physical, financial, and cultural obstacles. In addition to reducing possible barriers, psychologists working with the elderly are encouraged to operate within a multidisciplinary approach, working closely with other care providers, such as the primary care physician, a case manager, or a concerned family member. A competent geropsychologist must tolerate, understand, and strive to effectively negotiate interpersonal conflict and differences within or between older patients, families, and team members. Creating a trusting relationship with the client may be more easily facilitated if the person has confidence in the network of those providing care.

Self-Reflective Anti-Ageist Biases Competency

A competent geropsychologist should practice self-reflection, demonstrating awareness of personal biases, assumptions, stereotypes, and potential discomfort in working with older adults, particularly those whose backgrounds are different from that of the psychologist. Personal awareness is a must, as geropsychologists "recognize how their attitudes and beliefs about aging and about older individuals may be relevant to their assessment and treatment of older adults" (Knight et al., 2009, p. 212). That is, awareness of their own biases, and even possible ageism, is of significance, as competent geropsychologists should demonstrate self-awareness and ability to recognize differences between their own and the patient's values, attitudes, assumptions, hopes, and fears related to aging, caregiving, illness, disability, social supports, medical care, dying, and grief.

In a youth-oriented society, aging may carry a negative connotation for many trainees. Ageism, prejudice, or discrimination based on an individual's age can be subtle and are often manifested in negative views of aging held unintentionally, even by psychologists interested in working with older adults. One such stereotype is that all older adults are the same, with homogeneity occurring simultaneously with aging. Myths of the aging experience also include erroneous beliefs that older adults are rigid, sickly, and frail; cognitively impaired; and dependent upon others. However, existing literature clearly refutes these stereotypes within an aging population, and supervisors and trainees alike must strive to combat ageist misperceptions. A competent geropsychologist should initiate consultation with appropriate sources as needed to address specific areas of concern in regard to any potential for personal biases or prejudices.

Supervisors must not only model nonageist attitudes toward older adults but also be willing to confront those in training when they engage in ageist practices. For example, a therapist who in the course of individual therapy is willing to confront a 20-year-old client about her destructive behavior but not an 80-year-old woman about her equally destructive behavior may unintentionally be expressing ageist therapeutic interactions and possibly harming the older client. When presented with the possibility of treating someone differently because of his or her age, many therapists in training are willing to explore their own biases and perhaps are able to identify that they worry about their own age (What do I know about what it's like being 80?) or societal influences (She looks like a grandmother. She wouldn't abuse alcohol, would she?).

Countertransference

Distortions can occur in the therapeutic relationship, both from the client toward the therapist (transference), and from the therapist toward the client (countertransference). Psychologists must be aware of the possibility for these unconscious misrepresentations or reactions to the older client, possibly stemming from experiences in previous significant relationships or intrapersonal existential issues that might be stimulated when working with late-life individuals.

It is well known that therapists treating clients who are demographically different from themselves experience additional strain in the therapeutic process (Spiegel, 1965). This most likely includes younger trainees or psychologists who are working with those who are in comparison significantly advanced in age. Similar to ethnocultural transference which is based on a client-therapist dyad with each from differing ethnic backgrounds

(Comas-Diaz & Jacobsen, 1991, 1995), a younger therapist and older adult client dyad comprises unique processes and dynamics with the potential to hinder core therapeutic issues. For example, there may be a therapist's "denial of ethnocultural differences," in this case the belief that everyone over 70 is the same. The "clinical anthropologist syndrome" may also occur, as the younger therapist is excessively interested in the client's culture, with an over-zealous curiosity of what it is like to be 102 years of age or near death. Or, the younger therapist may experience increased "guilt and pity" for the older patient, feeling sorry for the 80-year-old with chronic back pain, limited finances, and loss of family members.

Based on the psychodynamic concept of countertransference, therapists may have views, either negative or overly positive, of older adults stemming from their own relationships with their parents, grandparents, or older relatives. For example, having memories of one's stereotypical domesticated gray-haired, loving, and sweet grandmother who made cookies throughout one's childhood could potentially influence the decision to complete a neuropsychological evaluation of an older female client who presents as being kindly and gentle, yet is estranged from her family and continues to experience periods of extreme agitation and episodes of memory loss. Or, watching one's parents act in a very parental or controlling way with their own aging parents could conceivably impact the therapeutic approach with an aging couple who come to therapy to explore their decisions about future living arrangements and care.

Clinicians working with older adults also must be aware of the existential nature of their work, as a competent geropsychologist is aware of the impact of advanced illness, caregiving, dying, and death on family members and caregivers, as well as the effect these issues have on one's self. The aging process and eventual death is something that becomes relevant at some point for everyone. Yalom (2008) began his most recent book about human reaction to death highlighting this very issue, as he wrote, "Self-awareness is a supreme gift, a treasure as precious as life," following with, "Our existence is forever shadowed by the knowledge that we will grow, blossom, and inevitably, diminish and die" (p. 1).

Geropsychology is one area of specialization with a greater potential for client deaths, as working with a late-life population increases the likelihood that clients will die. Competent geropsychologists should monitor internal thoughts and feelings that may influence their professional behavior, and adjust their behavior accordingly in order to focus on needs of the patient, family, and treatment team. There should be an introspective awareness that regardless of countless experiences or even familiarity, the exposure to ongoing suffering and the end of life can also provide its own distress. Basing the title of his book on this concept, Yalom (2008) wrote, "It's not easy to live every moment wholly aware of death. It's like trying to stare the sun in the face: you can stand only so much of it" (p. 5).

Supervisors of those learning to work with older adults must remain sensitive to this aspect of working with this population and help trainees to be aware and process their unique reactions to client death (Knight, 2004). Just as competent geropsychologists must be cognizant of the differences between normal grief reactions and complicated grief in older adults, they too must be introspective regarding their own reactions to death and their overall emotional well-being.

Business Practice in Professional Geropsychology

Perhaps one of the most ignored areas within the teaching of geropsychology concerns the business aspects of the profession (Hartman-Stein, 2006). Although much has been written about the clinical skills, ethics, and required knowledge for working with older adults, little attention has been given to the topic of the foundational competencies for business, even though it is clear that a competent geropsychologist should implement appropriate business practices. Business information in geropsychology is unfortunately often gained the hard way by trial and error when an experienced psychologist in an already developed practice decides to serve an additional population or branch out into a new and diverse setting, or when a recently licensed psychologist with some training in geropsychology decides to enter private practice. Geropsychology programs, as well as individual supervisors, will benefit students as well as the profession with increased attention to the business piece of geropsychology.

Just as general clinical skills apply to geropsychology clinical and assessment skills, a general business approach may also be useful as a beginning step for business practice in geropsychology. Thus, those working with older adults may benefit from general resources (e.g., Barnett & Henshaw, 2003; Walfish & Barnett, 2009) that prepare one for the business of private practice. Pope and Vasquez (2005) offer a wealth of strategies for those just beginning a practice, as well as for those who want to expand, redirect, or strengthen their current business.

Although these three resources are infinitely valuable, they do not include specifics for those wanting to establish an older adult specialty practice or include older adults in their general practice. In a perusal of 10 of the most commonly used books on clinical geropsychology and mental health for the aging, only one addressed the business side of a geropsychology practice. In *Psychotherapy for Depression in Older Adults* edited by Qualls and Knight (2006), Hartman-Stein (2006) summarized lessons she learned while writing articles for the National Psychologist and through her own self-managed practice. In the chapter appropriately entitled "The Basics of Building and Managing a Geropsychology Practice," she highlighted practical points for having a successful "niche practice" in geropsychology by expanding on three prominent business rules: "Know the business, know the market, and know the customer" (p. 229).

Those interested in working with older adults must be aware that clinical opportunities present themselves in a number of settings and activities, and a competent geropsychologist should be prepared for a variety of models for aging services delivery, demonstrating flexibility in professional roles to adapt to the realities of work in various aging or health care systems. These include direct services to outpatient populations, many of which have been described in previous chapters including psychotherapy, behavior modification, assessment, neuropsychological evaluation, cognitive retraining, group therapy, and facilitation of support groups. Psychologists may also want to provide services such as employee training and family member education.

Marketing is especially important to the clinician who decides to build a private practice specializing in older adults. Success may be increased by identifying a subspecialty area, such as assessment, neuropsychology, individual psychotherapy, group psychotherapy, consultation, or training. Targeting specific settings, such as long-term care or outpatient psychotherapy services, through alignment with a primary care doctor will also be useful. Networking with other health care professionals is an absolute must, as it will be helpful to identify individuals from related fields who specialize in geriatrics, such as physicians, nurse practitioners, physician assistants, and occupational/physical therapists. Developing marketing tools such as brochures or handouts is also beneficial for practice building.

MEDICARE

A competent geropsychologist should have a comprehensive understanding of Medicare, Medicaid, and other insurance coverage for diagnostic conditions and health and mental health care services for older adults. Medicare is the universal health care system, or federal insurance program, for Americans 65 years and older regardless of income, as well as for younger persons with disabilities and special needs. This is different from Medicaid, which is an assistance program that serves low-income people of every age. Medicaid is a federal-state program, and varies by state. However, in general, Medicaid beneficiaries usually pay no part of costs for covered medical expenses. The Centers for Medicare & Medicaid (CMS; www.cms. hhs.gov/) is the U.S. federal agency that administers Medicare and Medicaid. Medicare benefits include Part A (hospitalization), and Part B, which is the component that covers the costs of eligible professional services from health care providers such as psychologists and physicians, as well as other outpatient hospital care and medical services not requiring hospitalization, including home health care, durable medical equipment, physical therapy, x-ray and diagnostic tests. Medicare Part A is provided free of charge once individuals turn age 65 or older and they or their spouse worked and paid Medicare taxes for at least 10 years. Part B is optional, and beneficiaries pay a monthly premium.

Another option for older adults is Medicare Part C, which combines Medicare Parts A and B, with the main difference being that the policy is provided through private insurance companies approved by Medicare to offer this type of coverage. Part C plans include programs such as preferred provider organization (PPOs), health maintenance organizations (HMOs), and private fee-for-service (PFFS). The majority of these plans include pre-scription medication coverage. Medicare Part D is the most recent addition to Medicare coverage and is the prescription drug coverage insurance that is provided by private companies approved by Medicare. Part D was designed to help people with Medicare to lower their prescription drug costs and to protect against future costs.

Medicare Part B will be of most interest for the majority of psychologists, as Part B reimburses health care providers on a fee-for-service basis—which is how the majority of psychologists are currently reimbursed for their services to Medicare beneficiaries. Historically, Medicare has reimbursed psychological services at 50% of the fee, with the older adult being responsible for the co-pay. However, in July of 2008 Congress provided for Medicare coinsurance parity for Medicare patients when it enacted the Medicare Improvements for Patients and Providers Act (MIPPA). Under MIPPA, mental health services are paid at the same rate as other medical services, and are eligible for a 80%–20% split in coinsurance by 2014, with the phase-in to coinsurance parity for outpatient mental health services scheduled to begin in January 2010.

A competent geropsychologist should consistently be able to provide appropriate diagnostic and procedure coding for psychological services rendered. Although a majority of providers will utilize individual psychotherapy and testing codes for those with mental health diagnoses, a successful advancement for psychology came in January of 2002, when the codes for Health and Behavior assessment and intervention services (e.g., H & B codes) were able to be applied to behavioral, social, and psychophysiological procedures for the prevention, treatment, or management of physical health problems. Since then, psychologists have been able to bill for services provided to patients who have a physical health diagnosis, thus allowing a blend of physical and psychological services delivery. Services provided through H & B codes are reimbursed at the 80% level. Through engaging in a comprehensive approach to patient care, the H & B codes pertain to psychological intervention allowing clients to improve their health and functioning in a multitude of ways. For example, psychologists may focus on helping clients to engage in behaviors that help promote their health through encouraging compliance with treatment or providing motivation for various prescribed treatments. Psychologists may facilitate patient adjustment to their physical illness or address behavior that keeps patients from effectively engaging in treatment. Some of the H & B services involve circumstances and behaviors related to food and eating, where a psychologist can help to refine the dietary regimen to make it more palatable to the patient. H & B codes are also utilized in some circumstances where due to cognitive impairment, verbal psychotherapy is not an option, but yet there are significant psychological contributions that will facilitate recovery or rehabilitation.

Although Medicare covers a number of psychological and health-related services, there are significant regulations, policies, and requirements. Essential billing tools for the psychologist include CPT Code Book, ICD-9-CM Book, and Medicare or Private Insurance Carrier's Coverage Policy (Moore & Georgoulakis, 2008). A competent geropsychologist must stay abreast of the current system and be willing to change with mandated updates, utilizing resources such as professional newsletters and e-mail forums. It is the clinician's responsibility to be aware of all federal policy as well as the rules and regulations of all local or regional carriers that CMS contracts with to cover each of the states. A Local Coverage Determination (LCD) is a decision by a regional carrier on whether to cover a particular service on an intermediary-wide or carrier-wide basis, and must not contradict federal policy; but it can provide additional specificity or added requirements. Because ignorance is not an excuse, providers may be at risk for abuse, which "involves incidents or practices that are not medically necessary as defined by Medicare Guidelines or are inconsistent with accepted sound medical, business or fiscal practices"

(Georgoulakis, 2008). Abuse can be identified when individuals intentionally follow practices that result in unnecessary Medicare program costs. Abusive practices may develop into fraud and be prosecuted as such (Georgoulakis, 2008). APA provided the "Medicare Local Medical Review Policies Tool Kit" at www.apa.org/pi/aging/lmrp/toolkit/ to further assist psychologists interested in understanding Medicare policy and guidelines.

Medical Necessity

It should be noted that Medicare reimburses only services that are "medically necessary." Treatment must be reasonable with an expectation of improvement; that is, interventions must be designed to reduce or control the patient's psychiatric symptoms, or at a minimum improve or maintain the patient's level of functioning. CMS requires that all covered psychological services and treatment be "expected to improve the health status or function of the patient," with documentation to support this. Definitions of "medical necessity" vary widely across health plans and are likely to encompass multiple factors and considerations—only one of which is a clinician's professional judgment. In the CMS glossary, medically necessary is defined as "Services or supplies that are proper and needed for diagnosis or treatment of the patient's medical condition; furnished for the diagnosis, direct care, and treatment of the patient's medical condition; meet standards of good medical practice; and are not mainly for the convenience of the patient, provider, or supplier." However, little more is offered in regard to the objective criteria included in this definition.

One source of insight into medical necessity as defined by CMS is a review paper entitled "Medicare Payments for 2003 Part B Mental Health Services: Medical Necessity, Documentation, and Coding" (Department of Health and Human Services, Office of Inspector General, 2007). Released in April of 2007, the report noted that medical reviewers determined that psychological services were not medically necessary based on (1) psychotherapy session being too long; (2) patient not being able to benefit from the psychotherapy; (3) number of sessions per week too frequent; and/or (4) no clinical problem documented in the record.

Documenting treatment and medical necessity is of utmost importance. That is, documentation is vital to providing good, consistent patient care, but it is also imperative for reimbursement purposes. Reimbursement for provided services is most frequently denied because of incorrect coding, poor or insufficient documentation, and not meeting criteria for medical necessity. A competent geropsychologist should utilize medical record documentation that is consistent with Medicare, Medicaid, HIPAA, and other federal, state, or local or organizational regulations, including appropriate documentation of medical necessity for services. Although there is no one accepted authority or criterion for documentation, at a minimum documentation should include target symptoms, goals of therapy, methods of monitoring outcome, and how the treatment is expected to improve the health status or the functioning of the patient (Georgoulakis, 2008). "For psychotherapy codes, documentation will almost always meet requirements if it includes date of service, time spent for the encounter face-to-face, type of therapeutic intervention (that is, insight oriented, supportive, behavior modification, interactive), target symptoms, progress toward achievement of treatment goals, diagnoses, and a legible signature" (American Psychiatric Association, 2008, p. 26).

A review of CMS and regional policies suggests that providers should document how the patient is able to

- benefit from treatment
- actively participate in psychotherapy
- show improvement

Additional areas to document include

- why patient instability continues to require treatment and/or ongoing rationale for continued treatment
- established treatment goals **and** an intervention
- assessment of patient response to the treatment
- treatment strategy explaining how the particular intervention is intended to help the patient

Providers may also want to include information regarding patient functioning, such as scores from the Mini-Mental State Examination (MMSE; Folstein, Folstein, & McHugh, 1975), Geriatric Depression Scale (GDS; Yesavage, 1988), Global Assessment of Functioning (GAF) scale (American Psychiatric Association, 1994) and Minimum Data Set (MDS), a CMS standardized assessment for facilitating care management in nursing homes. Additional documentation might include a specific stated reason for the original referral for psychological services, and collateral documentation such as nursing, social service, and primary care physician progress notes that document psychological symptoms, need for treatment, and the patient's ability to benefit from individual psychotherapy.

Assessing Geropsychology Competencies

As Qualls (1998) noted, "Failure to recognize the unique aspects of geropsychology practice creates a barrier to competent practice" (p. 26). Regardless of the timing of the training to work with older adults, a competent geropsychologist should demonstrate accurate self-evaluation of knowledge and skill competencies related to work with diverse older adults, including those with particular diagnoses or in care settings, and when needed, seek continuing education, training, supervision, and consultation to enhance geropsychology competencies related to practice. The Pikes Peak Geropsychology Knowledge and Skill Assessment Tool (CoPGTP, 2008) is a competency evaluation measure, providing ratings across levels (e.g., novice, intermediate, advanced, proficient, expert) for the knowledge domain and skill competency aspects of the Pikes Peak Model. As a point of reference, the tool notes that "graduate practica students would be expected to perform at Novice through Advanced levels, while Postdoctoral Fellows in Geropsychology would be expected to perform from Intermediate to Expert levels" (CoPGTP, 2008, p. 2). The assessment scale assumes that the acquisition of competency in geropsychology is developmental in nature and thus appropriate for both the graduate student in a specialized geropsychology program and the seasoned general practitioner attending continuing education workshops. The tool can be accessed at www.uccs.edu/~cpgtp/Pikes%2520Peak%2520Evaluation%2520Tool%25201.1.pdf.

Conclusions

Geropsychologists have ample opportunity to engage in the teaching, supervision, clinical, and business aspects of the profession. Undergraduate education is likely to expand, including additional courses throughout the curriculum, as well as increased offering of certificates or degreed programs for learners who choose to specialize in working with older adults. At the graduate level, the call for psychologists who are trained to work with older adults has continued to be issued. Even those clinicians who do not specialize in geropsychology most likely will encounter older adults in their work. Based on the Pike's Peak Model, an aspirational competency-based approach to professional psychology, including aspects of teaching, supervision, and business, is offered for those at any stage of their training, to further support the needed skills in geropsychology.

REFERENCES

Abbass, A. A., Hancock, J. T., Henderson, J., & Kisely, S. (2006). Short-term psychodynamic psychotherapies for common mental disorders. *Cochrane Database of Systematic Reviews, Issue 4*: CD004687

Abramson, T. A., Trejo, L., & Lai, D. W. L. (2002). Culture and mental health: Providing appropriate services for a diverse older population. *Generations, 26*, 21–27.

Adams, K. (2001). Depressive symptoms, depletion, or developmental change? Withdrawal, apathy, or lack of vigor in the Geriatric Depression Scale. *The Gerontologist, 41*, 768–777.

Administration on Aging. (2001). *Achieving cultural competence: A guidebook for providers of services to older Americans and their families.* Retrieved December 29, 2008, from www.aoa.gov/prof/adddiv/cultural/CC-guidebook.pdf.

Administration on Aging. (2008). *Older Americans 2000: Key indicators of well-being. Appendix A: Detailed tables.* Retrieved December 28, 2008, from http://www.agingstats.gov/agingstatsdotnet/Main_Site/Data/2008_Documents/tables/Tables.aspx.

Administration on Aging. (n.d.). *Guidelines for culturally and/or linguistically competent agencies.* Retrieved December 29, 2008, from www.aoa.gov/prof/adddive/progmod/addiv_progmod_section_two.asp.

Agency for Healthcare Research and Quality. (2002). *Focus on research: Disparities in healthcare.* Publication No. 02-m027.

Alexopoulos, R. C., Abrams, R. C., Young, C. A., & Shamoian, C. A. (1988). The Cornell Scale for Depression in Dementia. *Biological Psychiatry, 23*, 271–284.

Alexopoulos, G., Raue, P., & Areán, P. (2003). Problem-solving therapy versus supportive therapy in geriatric major depression with executive dysfunction. *American Journal of Geriatric Psychiatry, 11*(1), 46–52.

Alexopoulos, G. S., Katz, I. R., Bruce, M. L., Heo, M., Ten Have, T., Raue, P., et al. (2005). Remission in depressed geriatric primary care patients: A report from the PROSPECT study. *American Journal of Psychiatry, 162*(4), 718–724.

Allen, K. R., Blieszner, R., & Roberto, K. A. (2000). Families in the middle and later years: A review and critique of research in the 1990s. *Journal of Marriage and the Family, 62*, 911–926.

Alliance for Aging Research. (2002). *Medical never-never land: Ten reasons why America isn't ready for the coming age boom.* Washington, DC: Alliance for Aging Research.

Allport, G.(1937). *Personality: A psychological interpretation.* New York: Henry Holt & Company.

Alzheimer's Association. (2004). Research consent for cognitively impaired adults: Recommendations for institutional review boards and investigators. *Alzheimer Disease and Associated Disorders, 18*(3), 171.

American Bar Association Commission on Law and Aging, American Psychological Association (2005). *Assessment of older adults with diminished capacity: A handbook for lawyers.* Washington, DC: American Bar Association and American Psychological Association.

American Bar Association and American Psychological Association Assessment of Capacity in Older Adults Project Working Group. (2006). *Judicial determination of capacity of older adults in guardianship proceedings: A handbook for judges.* Washington DC: American Bar Association and American Psychological Association.

American Bar Association and American Psychological Association Assessment of Capacity in Older Adults Project Working Group. (2008). *Assessment of older adults with diminished capacity: A handbook for psychologists.* Washington, DC: American Bar Association and American Psychological Association.

American Geriatrics Society. (2004). *Doorway thoughts: Cross-cultural health care for older adults.* Sudbury, MA: Jones and Bartlett.

American Geriatrics Society, and Association of Directors of Geriatric Academic Programs. (2004). *Geriatric medicine. A clinical imperative for an aging population.* New York: Author.

American Geriatrics Society Core Writing Group of the Task Force on the Future of Geriatric Medicine. (2005). Caring for older Americans: The future of geriatric medicine. *Journal of the American Geriatrics Society, 53,* S245–S256.

American Psychiatric Association. (1994). *Diagnostic and statistical manual of mental disorders* (4th ed.). Washington, DC: Author.

American Psychiatric Association. (2008). Document, document, document. *Psychiatric News, 43,* 26. Retrieved March 15, 2009 from http://pn.psychiatryonline.org/cgi/content/full/.

American Psychological Association. (1997, December). *What practitioners should know about working with older adults.* Retrieved December 28, 2009, from www.apa.org/pi/aging/practitioners.pdf.

American Psychological Association. (1998). *Interprofessional health care services in primary care settings: Implications for the education and training of psychologists.* Retrieved December 10, 2008, from www.apa.org/ed/samhsa.pdf.

American Psychological Association. (2002a). *APA resolution on ageism.* Retrieved December 28, 2008, from www.apa.org/pi/aging/ageism.html.

American Psychological Association. (2002b). Ethical principles of psychologists and code of conduct. *American Psychologist, 57*(12), 1060–1073.

American Psychological Association. (2003). Guidelines for multicultural education, training, research, practice, and organizational change for psychologists. *American Psychologist, 58,* 377–402.

American Psychological Association. (2004). Guidelines for psychological practice with older adults. *American Psychologist, 59*(4), 236–260.

American Psychological Association, Committee on Aging. (2005). *Life plan for the life span for psychologists.* Washington, DC: Author.

American Psychological Association. (2006*). Task force on the assessment of competence in professional psychology: Final report.* Retrieved December 17, 2008, from www.apa.org/ed.comeptency_revised. pdf.

American Psychological Association, Presidential Task Force on Integrated Health Care for an Aging Population. (2008). *Blueprint for change: Achieving integrated health care for an aging population.* Washington, DC: American Psychological Association.

American Psychological Association, Multicultural Competency in Geropsychology Working Group and Committee on Aging. (2009). *Multicultural competency in geropsychology report.* Retrieved August 13, 2009, from http://www.apa.org/pi/aging/.

American Psychological Association Working Group on the Older Adult (N. Abeles, S. Cooley, I. M. Deitch, M. S. Harper, G. Hinrichsen, M. Lopez, & V. Molinari). (1997). *What practitioners should know about working with older adults.* Washington, DC: American Psychological Association . Also in *Professional Psychology: Research and Practice,* 1998, *29,* 413–427.

Amore, M., Tagariello, P., Laterza, C., & Savoia, E. M. (2007). Beyond nosography of depression in elderly. *Archives of Gerontology and Geriatrics, 44 Suppl 1,* 13–22.

An, J. S., & Cooney, T. M. (2006). Psychological well-being in mid to late life: The role of generativity development and parent-child relationships across the lifespan. *International Journal of Behavioral Development, 30,* 410–421.

Anderson, R. J., Freedland, K. E., Clouse, R. E., & Lustman, P. J. (2001). The prevalence of comorbid depression in adults with diabetes: A meta-analysis. *Diabetes Care, 24,* 1069–1078.

Areán, P. A., Alvidrez, J., Barrera, A., Robinson, G. S., & Hicks, S. (2002). Would older medical patients use psychological services? *The Gerontologist, 42,* 392–398.

Areán P. A., Ayalon, L., Hunkeler, E., Lin, E. H., Tang, L., Harpole, L., et al. (2005). Improving depression care for older, minority patients in primary care. *Medical Care, 43*(4), 381–390.

Areán, P., & Huh, T. (2006). Problem-solving therapy with older adults. *Psychotherapy for depression in older adults* (pp. 133–151). Hoboken, NJ: John Wiley & Sons Inc.

Areán, P. A., Perri, M. G., Nezu, A. M., Schein, R. L., Christopher, F., & Joseph, T. X. (1993). Comparative effectiveness of social problem-solving therapy and reminiscence therapy as treatments for depression in older adults. *Journal of Consulting and Clinical Psychology,* 61, 1003–1010.

Ariyo, A. A., Haan, M., Tangen, C. M., Rutledge, J. C., Cushman, M., Dobs, A., & Furberg, C. D. (2000). Depressive symptoms and risks of coronary heart disease and mortality in elderly Americans. *Circulation, 102*(15), 1773–1779.

Armstrong-Stassen, M. (2001). Reactions of older employees to organizational downsizing: The role of gender, job level, and time. *Journal of Gerontology: Psychological Sciences and Social Sciences, 56B,* 234–243.

Arredondo, P., & Perez, P. (2006). Historical perspectives on the multicultural guidelines and contemporary applications. *Professional Psychology: Research and Practice, 37,* 1–5.

Association of Psychology Postdoctoral and Internship Centers. (2008). *APPIC online directory: Search the directory online.* Retrieved from www.appic.org/directory/search_dol_internships.asp

Atchley, R. C. (1989). A continuity theory of normal aging. *The Gerontologist, 29,* 183–190.

Aulisio, M. P., Arnold, R. M., & Youngner, S. J. (2000). Health care ethics consultation: Nature, goals, and competencies. A position paper from the society for health and human values-society for bioethics consultation task force on standards for bioethics consultation. *Annals of Internal Medicine, 133,* 59–69.

Ayers, C., Sorrell, J., Thorp, S., & Wetherell, J. (2007, March). Evidence-based psychological treatments for late-life anxiety. *Psychology and Aging,* 22(1), 8–17.

Back, M. F. & Huak, C.Y. (2005). Family centred decision making and non-disclosure of diagnosis in a South East Asian oncology practice. *Psycho-Oncology, 14*(12), 1052–1059.

Baltes, M. N. (1996). *The many faces of dependency in old age.* New York: Cambridge University Press.

Baltes, P. B., & Baltes, M. M. (1990). Psychological perspectives on successful aging: The model of selective optimization with compensation. In P. B. Baltes & M. M. Baltes (Eds.), *Successful aging: Perspectives from the behavioral sciences* (pp. 1–34). New York: Cambridge University Press.

Baltes, P. B., & Graf, P. (1996). Psychological aspects of aging: Facts and frontiers In D. Magnusson (Ed.), *The lifespan development of individuals: Behavioral, neurobiological, and psychosocial perspectives* (pp. 427–460). New York: Cambridge University Press.

Baltes, P., Lindenberger, U., & Staudinger, U. (2006). Life Span Theory in Developmental Psychology. *Handbook of child psychology (6th ed.): Vol 1, Theoretical models of human development* (pp. 569–664). Hoboken, NJ: John Wiley & Sons Inc.

Baltes, P. B., Staudinger, U. M., & Linderberger, U. (1999). Lifespan psychology: Theory and application to intellectual functioning. *Annual Review of Psychology, 51,* 471–507.

Banks, M. E. (2008). Women with disabilities: Cultural competence in rehabilitation psychology. *Disability and Rehabilitation, 30,* 184–190.

Banks, M. E., Buki, L., Gallardo, M. E., & Yee, B. W. (2007). Integrative healthcare and marginalized populations. In I. Serlin (Series Ed.) and M. A. DiCowden (Vol. Ed.), *Humanizing healthcare: A handbook for healthcare integration: Vol 1. Mind–body medicine* (pp. 147–173). Westport, CT: Greenwood.

Barnett, J. E., & Henshaw, E. (2003). Training to begin a private practice. In M. Prinstein, J. Mitchell, & M. D. Patterson (Eds.), *The portable mentor: Expert guide to a successful career in psychology* (pp. 145–156). New York: Kluwer Academic/Plenum.

Bartels, S. J. (2003). Improving the system of care for older adults with mental illness in the United States: Findings and recommendations for the President's New Freedom Commission on Mental Health. *American Journal of Geriatric Psychiatry, 11*(5), 486–497.

Bartels, S. J., Coakley, E. H., Zubritsky, C., Ware, J. H., Miles, K. M., Areán, P. A., et al. (2004). Improving access to geriatric mental health services: A randomized trial comparing treatment engagement with integrated versus enhanced referral care for depression, anxiety, and at-risk alcohol use. *American Journal of Psychiatry, 161,* 1455–1462.

Bass, J., Neugebauer, R., Clougherty, K. F., Verdeli, H., Wickramarante, P., Ndogoni, L., et al. (2006). Group interpersonal psychotherapy for depression in rural Uganda: 6-month outcomes: Randomised controlled trial. *British Journal of Psychiatry, 188,* 567–573.

Beach, M. C., Price, E. G., Gary, T., Robinson, K. A., Gozu, A., Palacio, A., et al. (2005). Cultural competence: A systematic review of healthcare provider educational interventions. *Medical Care, 43,* 356–373.

Beauchamp, T. L., & Childress, J. F. (2001). *Principles of biomedical ethics* (5th ed.). Oxford: Oxford University Press.

Beck, J. G. (2008). Treating generalized anxiety in a community setting. In D. Gallagher-Thompson, A. M. Steffen, & L. W. Thompson (Eds.), *Handbook of behavioral and cognitive therapies with older adults* (pp. 18-32). New York, NY: Springer.

Beck, A. T., Rush, A. J., Shaw, B. F., & Emery, G. (1979). *Cognitive therapy of depression.* New York: Guilford.

Beekman, A. T., Geerlings, S. W., Deeg, D. J., Smit, J. H., Schoevers, R. S., de Beurs, E., et al. (2002). The natural history of late-life depression: A 6-year prospective study in the community. *Archives of General Psychiatry, 59*, 605–611.

Behnke, S. (2009, March). Ethics Rounds: A multicultural conference and summit, and inauguration. *Monitor on Psychology, 64*–65.

Bennett, K. M. (2005). Psychological wellbeing in later life: The longitudinal effects of marriage, widowhood and marital status change. *International Journal of Geriatric Psychiatry, 20*, 280–284.

Bennett, K. M., Smith, P. T., & Hughes, G. M. (2005). Coping, depressive feelings and gender differences in late life widowhood. *Aging and Mental Health, 9*, 348–353.

Berg, J. W., Appelbaum, P. S., Lidz, C. W., & Parker, L. S. (2001). *Informed consent: Legal theory and clinical practice*. New York: Oxford.

Bieliauskas, L. A. (2005). Neuropsychological assessment of geriatric driving competence. *Brain Injury, 19*(3), 221–226.

Birbeck, G. L., Zingmond, D. S., Cui, X., & Vickrey, B. G. (2006). Multispecialty stroke services in California hospitals are associated with reduced mortality. *Neurology, 66*(10), 1527–1532.

Birren, B. A., Stine-Morrow, E. (August, 1996). *The development of Division 20: Past and future perspectives*. Washington DC: American Psychological Association, Division 20.

Birren, J. E., & Schaie, K. W. (Eds.). (1977). *Handbook of the psychology of aging* (5th ed.). New York: Van Nostrand Reinhold.

Birrer, R. B., & Vemuri, S. P. (2004). Depression in later life: A diagnostic and therapeutic challenge. *American Family Physician, 69*, 2375–2382.

Bjelland, I., Dahl, A. A., Haug, T. T., & Neckelmann, D. (2002). The validity of the Hospital Anxiety and Depression Scale: An updated literature review. *Journal of Psychosomatic Research, 52*, 69–77.

Blackhall, L. J., Murphy, S. T., Frank, G., & Michel, V. (1995). Ethnicity and attitudes toward patient autonomy. *JAMA, 274*(10), 820–825.

Blanchard-Fields, F., & Hess, T. M. (1996). *Perspectives on cognitive change in adulthood and aging* (4th ed.). San Diego: Academic Press.

Blanchet, S., Belleville, S., & Peretz, I. (2006). Episodic encoding in normal aging: Attentional resources hypothesis extended to musical material. *Aging, Neuropsychology, and Cognition, 13*, 490–502.

Blazer, D. (2003). Depression in late life: Review and commentary. *Medicine and Science, 58A*, 249–265.

Blazer, D., Bachar, J., & Hughes, D. (1987). Major depression with melancholia: A comparison of middle-aged and elderly adults. *Journal of the American Geriatrics Society, 35*, 927–932.

Blieszner, R. (1994). *Doctoral programs in adult development and aging*. Washington, DC: American Psychological Association, Division 20.

Bogner, H. R., Morales, K. H., Post, E. P., & Bruce, M. L. (2007). Diabetes, depression, and death: A randomized controlled trial of a depression treatment program for older adults based in primary care (PROSPECT). *Diabetes Care, 30*(12), 3005–3010.

Bolton, P., Bass, J., Neugebauer, R., Verdeli, H., Clougherty, K.F., Wickramaratne, P .J., et al. (2003). A clinical trial of group interpersonal psychotherapy for depression in rural Uganda. *JAMA, 289*, 3117–3124.

Bonanno, G. A., Wortman, C. B., Lehman, D. R., Tweed, R. G., Haring, M., Sonnega, J., et al. (2002). Resilience to loss and chronic grief: A prospective study from preloss to 18-months postloss. *Journal of Personality and Social Psychology, 83*, 1150–1164.

Bonanno, G. A., Wortman, C. B., & Nesse, R. M. (2004). Prospective patterns of resilience and maladjustment during widowhood. *Psychology and Aging, 19*, 260–271.

Bond, M. (2006). Psychodynamic psychotherapy in the treatment of mood disorders. *Current Opinion in Psychiatry, 19*, 40–43.

Borsen, S. (1995). *Models in psychiatric settings.* Paper presented at VA Conference managing the geriatric patient with combined medical and psychiatric problems: Beyond "keep away." Menlo Park, CA.

Bourgeois, M. S., Schulz, R., Burgio, L., & Beach, S. (2002). Skills training for spouses of patients with Alzheimer's disease: Outcomes of an intervention study. *Journal of Clinical Geropsychology, 8,* 53–73.

Brenes, G.A., Wagener, P., & Stanley, M.A. (2008). Treatment of late-life generalized anxiety disorder in primary care settings. In D. Gallagher-Thompson, A.M. Steffen, & L.W. Thompson (Eds.), *Handbook of behavioral and cognitive therapies with older adults* (pp. 33–47). New York, NY: Springer.

Brennan, P. L., Schutte, K. K., & Moos, R. H. (2006). Long-term patterns and predictors of successful stressor resolution in later life. *International Journal of Stress Management, 13,* 253–272.

Brickman, A. M., Zimmerman, M. E., Paul, R. H., Grieve, S. M., Tate, D. F., Cohen, R. A., et al. (2006). Regional white matter and neuropsychological functioning across the adult lifespan. *Biological Psychiatry, 60,* 444–453.

Bronfenbrenner, U., & Morris, P. A. (2006). The bioecological model of human development. In W. Damon (Series Ed.) & R. M. Lerner (Vol. Ed.), *Handbook of child psychology: Vol. 1. Theoretical models of human development* (6th ed., pp. 793–828). New York: Wiley.

Brown, E. S., Khan, D. A., & Netjek, V. A. (1999). The psychiatric side effects of corticosteroids. *Annals of Allergy, Asthma, and Immunology, 83,* 495–504.

Bruce, M. L. (2002). Psychosocial risk factors for depressive disorders in late life. *Biological Psychiatry, 52,* 175–184.

Bruce, M. L., Ten Have, T. R., Reynolds, C.F., III, Katz, I. I., Schulberg, H. C., Mulsant, B. H., et al. (2004). Reducing suicidal ideation and depressive symptoms in depressed older primary care patients: A randomized controlled trial. *JAMA, 291,* 1081–1091.

Brummett, B. H., Babyak, M. A., Williams, R. B., Barefoot, J. C., Costa, P. T., & Siegler, I. C. (2006). NEO personality domains and gender predict levels and trends in body mass index over 14 years during midlife. *Journal of Research in Personality, 40,* 222–236.

Burck, R., & Lapidos, S. (2002). Ethics and cultures of care. In M. D. Mezey, C. K. Cassell, M. M. Bottrell, K. Hyer, J. L. Howe, & T. T. Fulmer (Eds.), *Ethical patient care: A casebook for geriatric health care teams* (pp. 41–66). Baltimore, MD: Johns Hopkins University Press.

Burgio, L. (1996). Interventions for the behavioral complications of Alzheimer's disease: Behavioral approaches. *International Journal of Psychogeriatrics, 1,* 45–52.

Burgio, L., Hardin, M., Sinnott, J., Janosky, J., & Hohman, M. (1995). Acceptability of behavioral treatments and pharmacotherapy for behaviorally disturbed older adults: Ratings of caregivers and relatives. *Journal of Clinical Geropsychology, 1*(1), 19–32.

Bush, S. S. (2008). *Geriatric mental health ethics: A casebook*. New York: Springer.

Callahan, C. M., Boustani, M. A., Unverzagt, F. W., Austrom, M. G., Damush, T. M., Perkins, A. J., et al. (2006). Effectiveness of collaborative care for older adults with Alzheimer's disease in primary care: A randomized controlled trial. *JAMA, 295,* 2148–2157.

Callahan, C. M., Hui, S. L., Nienaber, N. A., Musick, B. S., & Tierney, W. M. (1994). Longitudinal study of depression and health services use among elderly primary care patients. *Journal of the American Geriatrics Society, 42*(8), 833–838.

Callahan, C. M., Kroenke, K., Counsell, S. R., Hendrie, H. C., Perkins, A. J., Katon, W., et al. (2005). Treatment of depression improves physical functioning in older adults. *Journal of the American Geriatrics Society, 53*(3), 367–373.

Camp C. J., Foss J. W., Stevens A. B., Reichard C. C., McKitrick L. A., & O'Hanlon, A. M. (1993). Memory training in normal and demented elderly populations: The E-I-E-I-O model. *Experimental Aging Research, 19*(3), 277–290.

Cantor, M. D., & Pearlman, R. A. (2004). Advance care planning in long-term care facilities. *Journal of the Medical Directors Association, 5,* S72–80.

Carnelley, K. B., Wortman, C. B., Bolger, N., & Burke, C. T. (2006). The time course of grief reactions to spousal loss: Evidence from a national probability sample. *Journal of Personality and Social Psychology, 91,* 476–492.

Carney, R. M., & Freeland, K. E. (2008). Depression in patients with coronary heart disease. *American Journal of Medicine, 121*(11 Suppl 2), S20–S27.

Carpenter, B. D., Kissel, E. C., & Lee, M. M. (2007). Preferences and life evaluations of older adults with and without dementia: Reliability, stability, and proxy knowledge. *Psychology and Aging, 22*(3), 650–655.

Carpenter, B. D., Van Haitsma, K., Ruckdeschel, K., & Lawton, M. P. (2000). The psychosocial preferences of older adults: A pilot examination of content and structure. *The Gerontologist, 40*(3), 335–348.

Carreira, K., Miller, M. D., Frank, E., Houck, P. R., Morse, J. Q., Dew, M. A., et al. (2008). A controlled evaluation of monthly maintenance Interpersonal Psychotherapy in late-life depression with varying levels of cognitive function. *International Journal of Geriatric Psychiatry, 23,* 1110–1113.

Carson, A. J., MacHale, S., Allen, K., Lawrie, S. M., Dennis, M., House, A., et al. (2000). Depression after stroke and lesion location: A systematic review. *Lancet, 356,* 122–126.

Carstensen, L. L. (1991). Socioemotional and selectivity theory: Social activity in the life span context. *Annual Review of Gerontology and Geriatrics, 11,* 195–217.

Cassel, C. K., Mezey, M. D., & Bottrell, M. M. (2002). An introduction to bioethics as it relates to teams and geriatrics. In M. D. Mezey, C. K. Cassel, M. M. Bottrell, K. Hyer, J. L. Howe, & T. T. Fulmer (Eds.), *Ethical patient care: A casebook for geriatric health care teams* (pp. 3–22). Baltimore, MD: Johns Hopkins University Press.

Cavanaugh, J. C., & Blanchard-Fields, F. (2006). *Adult development and aging* (5th ed.). Belmont, CA: Wadsworth/Thomson.

Centers for Disease Control and Prevention. (2007). *The state of aging and health in America.* Whitehouse Station, NJ: Merck Company Foundation.

Chambless, D. L., & Ollendick, T. H. (2001). Empirically supported psychological interventions: Controversies and evidence. *Annual Review of Psychology, 52,* 685–716.

Charney, D. S., Reynolds, C. F., III, Lewis, L., Lebowitz, B. D., Sunderland, T., Alexopoulos, G. S., et al. (2003). Depression and Bipolar Support Alliance consensus statement on the unmet needs in diagnosis and treatment of mood disorders in late life. *Archives of General Psychiatry, 60,* 664–672.

Chen, H., Coakley, E. H., Cheal, K., Maxwell, J., Costantino, G., Krahn, D. D., et al. (2006). Satisfaction with mental health services in older primary care patients. *American Journal of Geriatric Psychiatry, 14,* 371–379.

Chichin, E. R., & Mezey, M. D. (2002). Professional attitudes toward end-of-life decision making. In M. D. Mezey, C. K. Cassell, M. M. Bottrell, K. Hyer, J. L. Howe, & T. T. Fulmer (Eds.), *Ethical patient care: A casebook for geriatric health care teams* (pp. 67–80). Baltimore, MD: Johns Hopkins University Press.

Chodosh, J., Kado, D. M., Seeman, T. E., & Karlamangla, A. S. (2007). Depressive symptoms as a predictor of cognitive decline: MacArthur Studies of Successful Aging. *American Journal of Geriatric Psychiatry, 55* (Suppl. 2), S403–408.

Ciechanowski, P., Wagner, E., Schmaling, K., Schwartz, S., Williams, B., Diehr, P., et al. (2004). Community-integrated home-based depression treatment in older adults: A randomized control trial. *JAMA, 291,* 1569–1577.

Cipher, D., Clifford, P., & Roper, K. (2007). The effectiveness of geropsychological treatment in improving pain, depression, behavioral disturbances, functional disability, and health care utilization in long-term care. *Clinical Gerontologist, 30*(3), 23–40.

Clayman, M. L., Roter, D., Wissow, L. S., & Bandeen-Roche, K. (2005). Autonomy-related behaviors of patient companions and their effect on decision-making activity in geriatric primary care visits. *Social Science and Medicine, 60*(7), 1583–1591.

Clifford, P. A., Cipher, D. J., Roper, K. D., Snow, A. L., & Molinari, V. (2008). Cognitive-behavioral pain management interventions for long-term care residents with physical and cognitive disabilities. In D. Gallagher-Thompson, A. M. Steffen, & L. W. Thompson (Eds.), *Handbook of behavioral and cognitive therapies with older adults* (pp. 76–101). New York: Springer.

Cohen-Mansfield, J. (2001). Non-pharmacologic interventions for inappropriate behaviors in dementia: A review, summary, and critique. *American Journal of Geriatric Psychiatry, 9*(4), 361–381.

Comas-Diaz, L., & Jacobsen, F. M. (1991) Ethnocultural transference and countertransference in the therapeutic dyad. *American Journal of Orthopsychiatry, 61,* 392–402.

Comas-Diaz, L., & Jacobsen, F. M. (1995). The therapist of color and the white patient dyad: Contradictions and recognitions. *Cultural Diversity and Mental Health, 1,* 93–106.

Committee on Quality Health Care in America. (2001). *Crossing the quality chasm: A new health system for the 21st century.* Washington, DC: National Academy Press.

Cook, A. J. (1998). Cognitive-behavioral pain management for elderly nursing home residents. *Journal of Gerontology: Psychological Sciences and Social Sciences, 53B,* 51–59.

Cook, K. G., Nau, S. D., & Lichstein, K. L. (2005). Behavioral treatment of late-life insomnia. In L. VandeCreek (Ed.), *Innovations in clinical practice: Focus on adults* (pp. 65–81). Sarasota, FL: Professional Resource Press.

Council of Professional Geropsychology Training Programs. (2008, Version 1.0). *Pikes Peak Geropsychology Knowledge and Skill Assessment Tool.* Retrieved March 11, 2009, from www.uccs.edu/~cpgtp/Pikes_Peak_Evaluation_Tool_1.0.pdf.

Coverdale, J., McCullough, L. B., Molinari, V., & Workman, R. (2006). Ethically justified clinical strategies for promoting geriatric assent. *International Journal of Geriatric Psychiatry, 21*(2), 151–157.

Crewe, S. E. (2004). Ethnogerontology: Preparing culturally competent social workers for the diverse facing of aging. *Journal of Gerontological Social Work, 43,* 45–58.

Cronbach, L. J. (1971). Test validation. In R. L. Thorndike (Ed.), *Educational measurement* (2nd ed., pp. 443–507). Washington, DC: American Council on Education.

Cronbach, L. J., & Meehl, P. E. (1955). Construct validity in psychological tests. *Psychological Bulletin, 52,* 281-302.

Cullen, B., O'Neill, B., Evans, J. J., Coen, R. F., & Lawlor, B.A. (2007). A review of screening tests for cognitive impairment. *Journal of Neurology, Neurosurgery, & Psychiatry, 78,* 790–799.

Curtis, E. F., & Dreachslin, J. L. (2008). Integrative literature review: Diversity management interventions and organizational performance: A synthesis of current literature. *Human Resource Development Review, 7,* 107–134.

Dafer, R., Rao, M., Shareef, A., & Sharma, A. (2008). Poststroke depression. *Top Stroke Rehabilitation, 15,* 13–21.

Daniel, J. H., Roysircar, G., Abeles, N., & Boyd, C. (2004). Individual and cultural diversity competency: Focus on the therapist. *Journal of Clinical Psychology, 60,* 755–770.

Davis, H. P., Trussell, L. H., & Klebe, K. J. (2001). A ten-year longitudinal examination of repetition priming, incidental recall, free recall, and recognition in young and elderly. *Brain and Cognition, 46,* 99–104.

Degrazia, D. (1999). Advance directives, dementia, and "the someone else problem." *Bioethics, 13,* 373–391.

Delano-Wood, L., & Abeles, N. (2005). Late-life depression: Detection, risk reduction, and somatic intervention. *Clinical Psychology: Science and Practice, 12,* 207–217.

Department of Health and Human Services, Office of Inspector General. (2007). *Medicare payment for 2003 Part B mental health services: Medical necessity, documentation, and coding title of document.* Retrieved May 28, 2009 from http://oig.hhs.gov/oei/reports/oei-09-04-00220.pdf

DeVries, H. M. (2005). Clinical geropsychology training in generalist doctoral programs. *Gerontology and Geriatrics Education, 25,* 5–20.

Dobson, K., Backs-Dermott, B., & Dozois, D. (2000). Cognitive and cognitive behavioral therapies. In C. R. Snyder & R. E. Ingram (Eds.), *Handbook of psychological change: Psychotherapy processes & practices for the 21st century* (pp. 409–428). Hoboken, NJ: John Wiley & Sons Inc.

Doolittle, N. O., & Herrick, C. A. (1992). Ethics in aging: A decision making paradigm. *Educational Gerontology, 18,* 395–408.

Duberstein, P. R., & Conwell, Y. (2000). Suicide. In S. K. Whitbourne (Ed.), *Psychopathology in later life* (pp. 245–276). New York: Wiley.

Duffy, M. (1992). Challenges in geriatric psychotherapy. *Individual Psychology, 48,* 432–444.

Duffy, M. (Ed.) (1999). *Handbook of counseling and psychotherapy with older adults.* New York: Wiley Press

Duffy, M. (2004). Curative factors in work with older adults. In D. P. Charman (Ed.), *Core processes in brief psychodynamic psychotherapy: Advancing effective process* (pp. 361–381). Hillsdale, N.J.: Lawrence Erlbaum.

Duffy, M., & Morales, P. (1997). Supervision of psychotherapy with older patients. In C. E. Watkins (Ed.), *Handbook of psychotherapy supervision* (pp. 366–380). New York: John Wiley.

Duner, A., & Nordstrom, M. (2005). Intentions and strategies among elderly people: Coping in everyday life. *Journal of Aging Studies, 19*, 437–451.

Dupree, L. W., Watson, M. A., & Schneider, M. G. (2005). Preferences for mental health care: A comparison of older African Americans and older Caucasians. *Journal of Applied Gerontology, 24*, 196–210.

Dura, J. R., Stukenberg, K. W., & Kiecolt-Glaser, J. K. (1990). Chronic stress and depressive disorders in older adults. *Journal of Abnormal Psychology, 99*, 284–290.

D'Zurilla, T. (1986). *Problem solving therapy: A social competence approach to clinical intervention.* New York: Springer Publishing Company.

D'Zurilla, T., & Goldfried, M. (1971, August). Problem solving and behavior modification. *Journal of Abnormal Psychology, 78*(1), 107–126.

Eaton, W. W., Smith, C., Ybarra, M, Muntaner, C., & Tien, A. (2004). Center for Epidemiological Studies Depression Scale: Review and re-vision (CESD and CESD-R). In E. Maruish (Ed.), *The use of psychological testing for treatment planning and outcomes assessment: Volume 3. Instruments for adults* (pp. 363–377). Mahwah, NJ: Erlbaum.

Ecklund, K., & Johnson, W. B. (2007). Toward cultural competence in child intake assessments. *Professional Psychology: Research and Practice, 38*, 356–362.

Edelstein, B., Martin, R., & Koven, L. (2003). Assessment in geriatric settings. In J. R. Graham & J. A. Naglieri (Eds.), *Comprehensive handbook of psychology: Vol. 10: Assessment psychology* (pp. 389–417). New York: Wiley.

Edelstein, B., Woodhead, E., Segal, D., Heisel, M., Bower, E., Lowery, A., et al. (2008). Older adult psychological assessment: Current instrument status and related considerations. *Clinical Gerontologist, 31*, 1–35.

Eisdorfer, C., & Lawton, M. P. (Eds.). (1973). *The psychology of adult development and aging.* Washington, DC: American Psychological Association.

Emery, E., Karel, M., Konnert, C., Pachana, N., Laidlaw, K., & Knight, B. (2007). *Geropsychology training opportunities in the US, UK, Canada, and Australia: An international comparison.* Symposium presented at the annual meeting of the Gerontological Society of America, San Francisco, CA.

Erber, J. T. (2005). *Aging and older adulthood.* Belmont, CA: Wadsworth/Thomson Learning.

Erikson, E. H. (1963). *Childhood and society* (2nd ed.). New York: Norton.

Farrell, M. P., Schmitt, M. H., & Heinemann, G. D. (2001). Informal roles and the stages of interdisciplinary team development. *Journal of Interprofessional Care, 15*(3), 281–295.

Federal Interagency Forum on Aging-Related Statistics. (2008). Retrieved November 15, 2008, from http://agingstats.gov/agingstatsdotnet/Main_Site/Data/2008_Documents/Health_Status.aspx on.

Federal Interagency Forum on Aging-Related Statistics. (2008). *Older Americans 2008: Key indicators of well-being.* Washington, DC: U.S. Government Printing Office.

Feinberg, L. F., & Whitlatch, C. J. (2001). Are persons with cognitive impairment able to state consistent choices? *The Gerontologist, 41*(3), 374–382.

Ferrario, S. R., Cardillo, V., Vicario, F., Balzarini, E., & Zotti, A. M. (2004). Advanced cancer at home: Caregiving and bereavement. *Palliative Medicine, 18*, 129–136.

Ferraro, F. R. (2006). Teaching tips: Selective review of some recent (and not so recent) adulthood and aging texts. Retrieved November 20, 2008 from http://apadiv20.phhp.ufl.edu/Teachtips/Summer%202006%20Selective%20Review.pdf.

Field, N. P., Nichols, C., Holen, A., & Horowitz, M. J. (1999). The relation of continuing attachment to adjustment in conjugal bereavement. *Journal of Consulting and Clinical Psychology, 67,* 212–218.

Fiksenbaum, L. M., Greenglass, E. R., & Eaton, J. (2006). Perceived social support, hassles, and coping among the elderly. *Journal of Applied Gerontology, 25,* 17–30.

Fischer, G. S., Arnold, R. M., & Tulsky, J. A. (2000). Talking to the older adult about advance directives. *Death and Dying, 16,* 239–254.

Fiske, A., & O'Riley, A. A. (2008). Depression in late life. In J. Hunsley & E. J. Mash (Eds.), *A guide to assessments that work* (pp. 138–158). New York: Oxford University Press.

Flores, G. (2006). Language barriers in health care in the United States: Perspective. *New England Journal of Medicine, 355*(3), 229–231.

Folstein, M. F., Folstein, S. E., & McHugh, P. R. (1975). "Mini Mental State": A practical method of grading the cognitive state of patients for the clinician. *Journal of Psychiatric Research, 12(3),* 189–198.

Foos, P. W., & Clark, M. C. (2003). *Human aging.* Boston, MA: Allyn & Bacon.

Fox, E., Berkowitz, K. A., Chanko, B. L., & Powell, T. (2005). *Ethics consultation: Responding to ethics concerns in health care.* Washington, DC: National Center for Ethics in Health Care, Veterans Health Administration.

Frazer, D., Leicht, M. L., & Baker, M. D. (1996). Psychological manifestations of physical disease in the elderly. In L. Carstensen, B. Edelstein, & L. Dornbrand (Eds.). *The practical handbook of clinical gerontology* (pp. 217-238). Thousand Oaks, CA: Sage.

Fretz, B. R. (1993). Counseling psychology: A transformation for the third age. *Counseling Psychologist, 21,* 154–170.

Friedman, D., & Berger, D. L. (2004). Improving team structure and communication: A key to hospital efficiency. *Archives of General Surgery, 139,* 1194–1198.

Friedman, L., Benson, K., Noda, A., Zarcone, V., Wicks, D., O'Connell, K., et al. (2000, March). An actigraphic comparison of sleep restriction and sleep hygiene treatments for insomnia in older adults. *Journal of Geriatric Psychiatry and Neurology, 13*(1), 17–27.

Fulmer, T., Flaherty, E., & Hyer, K. (2003). The geriatric interdisciplinary team training (GITT) program. *Gerontology and Geriatrics Education, 24*(2), 3–12.

Fultz, N. H., Jenkins, K. R., Ostbye, T., Taylor, D. H. J., Kabeto, M. U., & Langa, K. M. (2005). The impact of own and spouse's urinary incontinence on depressive symptoms. *Social Science and Medicine, 60,* 2537–2548.

Gade, G., Venohr, I., Conner, D., McGrady, K., Beane, J., Richardson, R. H., et al. (2008). Impact of an inpatient palliative care team: A randomized control trial. *Journal of Palliative Medicine, 11*(2), 180–190.

Gallagher-Thompson, D., & Coon, D. (2007). Evidence-based psychological treatments for distress in family caregivers of older adults. *Psychology and Aging, 22*(1), 37–51.

Gallagher-Thompson, D., Dupart, T., Liu, W., Gray, H., Eto, T., & Thompson, L.W. (2008). Assessment and treatment issues in bereavement in later life. In K. Laidlaw & B. Knight (Eds.), *Handbook of emotional disorders in later life: Assessment and treatment* (pp. 287–307). New York, NY: Oxford.

Gallagher-Thompson, D., Futterman, A., Farberow, N., Thompson, L. W., & Peterson, J. (1993). The impact of spousal bereavement on older widows and widowers. In M. S. Stroebe, W. Stroebe, & R. O. Hansson (Eds.), *Handbook of bereavement* (pp. 227–239). Cambridge, UK: Cambridge University Press.

Gallagher-Thompson, D., Haley, W., Guy, D., Rupert, M., Arguelles, T., Zeiss, L. M., et al. (2003). Tailoring psychological interventions for ethnically diverse dementia caregivers. *Clinical Psychology: Science and Practice, 10*, 423–438.

Gallagher-Thompson, D., Hanley-Peterson, P., & Thompson, L. W. (1990). Maintenance of gains versus relapse following brief psychotherapy for depression. *Journal of Consulting and Clinical Psychology, 58*, 371–374.

Gallagher-Thompson, D., Lovett, S., Rose, J., McKibbin, C., Coon, D., Futterman, A., & Thompson, L. W. (2000). Impact of psychoeducational interventions on distressed family caregivers. *Journal of Clinical Geropsychology, 6*, 91–110.

Gallagher-Thompson, D. E., & Steffen, A. M. (1994). Comparative effects of cognitive-behavioral and brief psychodynamic psychotherapies for depressed family caregivers. *Journal of Consulting and Clinical Psychology, 62*, 543–549.

Gallo, J. J., Rebok, G. W., Tennsted, S., Wadley, V. G., & Horgas, A. (2003). Linking depressive symptoms and functional disability in late life. *Aging and Mental Health, 7*, 469–480.

Gallo, W. T., Bradley, E. H., Dubin, J. A., Jones, R. N., Falba, T. A., Teng, H. M., et al. (2006). The persistence of depressive symptoms in older workers who experience involuntary job loss: Results from the health and retirement survey. *Journal of Gerontology: Social Sciences, 61B*, S221–S228.

Ganguli, M., & Hendrie, H. C. (2005). Screening for cognitive impairment and depression in ethnically diverse older populations. *Alzheimer's Disease and Associated Disorders, 19*, 275–278.

Ganzini, L., Volicer, L., Nelson, W., & Derse, A. (2003). Pitfalls in assessment of decision-making capacity. *Psychosomatics: Journal of Consultation Liaison Psychiatry, 44*(3), 237–243.

Garb, H. (1984). The incremental validity of information used in personality assessment. *Clinical Psychology Review, 4*, 641–655.

Gass, K. A. (1989). Appraisal, coping, and resources: Markers associated with the health of aged widows and widowers. In D. A. Lund (Ed.), *Older bereaved spouses: Research and practical applications* (pp. 79–94). New York: Hemisphere.

Gatz, M., & Finkel, S. I. (1995). Education and training of mental health service providers. In M. Gatz (Ed.), *Emerging issues in mental health and aging* (pp. 282–302). Washington, DC: American Psychological Association.

Gatz, M., Fiske, A., Fox, L. S., Kaskie, B., Kasl-Godley, J. E., McCallum, T. J., et al. (1998). Empirically validated psychological treatments for older adults. *Journal of Mental Health and Aging, 41*, 9–46.

Gatz, M., Karel, M. J., & Wolkenstein, B. (1991). Survey of providers of psychological services to older adults. *Professional Psychology: Research and Practice, 22*(5), 413–415.

Gauthier, A., & Serber, M. (2005). *A need to transform the U.S. health care system: Improving access, quality, and efficiency.* New York: Commonwealth Fund.

Gazmararian, J. A., Baker, D. W., Williams, M. V., Parker, R. M., Scott, T. L., Green, D. C., et al. (1999). Health literacy among Medicare enrollees in a managed care organization. *JAMA, 281*, 545–551.

Geerlings, S. W., Beekman, A. T., Deeg, D. J., Twisk, J. W., & Van Tilburg, W. (2002). Duration and severity of depression predict mortality in older adults in the community. *Psychological Medicine, 32,* 609–618.

Gentry, W. D. (1977). *Geropsychology: A model of training and clinical service.* Cambridge, MA: Ballinger.

Georgoulakis, J. M. (2008, August). *Medicare participation, billing and fraud's red flags.* Presentation at the annual meeting of the American Psychological Association, Boston, MA.,

Geropsychology Knowledge and Skill Assessment Tool. Retrieved from www.uccs. edu/~cpgtp/Pikes%2520Peak%2520Evaluation%2520Tool%25201.1.pd.

Gibson, P. G., Powell, H., Coughlan, J., Wilson, A. J., Abramson, M., Haywood, P., et al. (2003). Self-management education and regular practitioner review for adults with asthma. *Cochrane Database of Systematic Reviews,* 1:CD001117.

Giger, J., Davidhizar, R. E., Purnell, L., Harden, J. T., Phillips, J., & Stickland, O. (2007). American Academy of Nursing Expert Panel Report: Developing cultural competence to eliminate health disparities in ethnic minorities and other vulnerable populations. *Journal of Transcultural Nursing, 18,* 95–102.

Gill, S. C., Butterworth, P., Rodgers, B., Anstey, K. J., Villamil, E., & Melzer, D. (2006). Mental health and the timing of men's retirement. *Social Psychiatry and Psychiatric Epidemiology, 41,* 933–954.

Gillick, M. (1995). Medical decision-making for the unbefriended nursing home resident. *Journal of Ethics, Law, and Aging, 1,* 87–92.

Golden, R., & Emery, E. (2007). *BRIGHTEN: An interdisciplinary "virtual" team to treat depression in primary care.* Symposium presented at the Annual Meeting of the Gerontological Society of America, San Francisco, CA.

Goldfarb, A. I. (1955). Psychotherapy of aged persons: IV. One aspect of the psychodynamics of the therapeutic situation with aged patients. *Psychoanalytic Review, 42,* 180–187.

Goode, T. D., & Sockalingam, S. (2000). Cultural competence: Developing policies to address the health care needs of culturally diverse clients. *Home Health Care Management and Practice, 12,* 49–55.

Gournellis, R., Lykouras, L., Fortos, A., Oulis, P., Roumbos, V., & Christodoulou, G. N. (2001). Psychotic (delusional) major depression in late life: A clinical study. *International Journal of Geriatric Psychiatry, 16,* 1085–1091.

Granholm, E., McQuaid, J., McClure, F., Auslander, L., Perivoliotis, D., Pedrelli, P., et al. (2005). A randomized, controlled trial of cognitive behavioral social skills training for middle-aged and older outpatients with chronic schizophrenia. *American Journal of Psychiatry, 162,* 520-529.

Granholm, E., McQuaid, J., McClure, F., Link, P., Perivoliotis, D., Gottlieb, J., et al. (2007, May). Randomized controlled trial of cognitive behavioral social skills training for older people with schizophrenia: 12-month follow-up. *Journal of Clinical Psychiatry, 68*(5), 730-737.

Greenwood, P. M. (2007). Functional plasticity in cognitive aging: Review and hypothesis. *Neuropsychology, 21,* 657–673.

Griffin, B. P., & Grunes, J. M. (1990). A developmental approach to psychoanalytic psychotherapy with the aged. In R. A. Nemiroff & C. A. Colarruso (Eds.), *New dimensions in adult development* (pp. 267–283). New York: Basic Books.

Grisso, T. (1986). *Evaluating competencies.* New York: Plenum.

Grisso, T. (2003). *Evaluating competencies: Forensic assessments and instruments* (2nd ed.). New York: Kluwer Academic.

Grisso, T., & Applebaum, T. S. (1989). *Assessing competence to consent to treatment: A guide for physicians and other health professionals.* New York: Oxford University Press.

Gurland, B. J., Cross, P. S., & Katz, S. (1996). Epidemiological perspectives on opportunities for treatment of depression. *American Journal of Geriatric Psychiatry, 4 (Suppl. 1),* S7–S13.

Gutmann, D. L. (1992). Toward a dynamic geropsychology. In J. W. Barron, M. N. Eagle, & D. L. Wolitsky, *Interface of psychoanalysis and psychology* (pp. 284–296). Washington, DC: American Psychological Association.

Haber, D. (2005). Cultural diversity among older adults: Addressing health education. *Educational Gerontology, 31,* 683–697.

Hajjar, E. R., Cafiero, A. C., & Hanlon, J. T. (2007). Polypharmacy in elderly patients. *American Journal of Geriatric Pharmacotherapy, 5,* 345–351.

Haley, W. E., Allen, R. S., Reynolds, S., Chen, H., Burton, A., & Gallagher-Thompson, D. (2002). Family issues in end-of-life decision making and end-of-life care. *American Behavioral Scientist, 46*(2), 284–298.

Halpain, M. C., Harris, M. J., McClure, F. S., & Jeste, D. V. (1999). Training in geriatric mental health: Needs and strategies. *Psychiatric Services. 50*(9), 1205–1208.

Hammes, B. J., & Rooney, B. L. (1998). Death and end-of-life planning in one midwestern community. *Archives of Internal Medicine, 158,* 383–390.

Hansen, N. D., Pepitone-Arreola-Rockwell, F., & Greene, A. F. (2000). Multicultural competence: Criteria and case examples. *Professional Psychology: Research and Practice, 31,* 652–660.

Hansen, N. D., Randazzo, K. V., Schwartz, A., Marshall, M., Kalis, D., Frazier, R., et al. (2006). Do we practice what we preach? An exploratory survey of multicultural psychotherapy competencies. *Professional Psychology: Research and Practice, 37,* 66–74.

Hanson, S. L., Kerkhoff, T. R., & Bush, S. S. (2005). *Health care ethics for psychologists: A casebook.* Washington, DC: American Psychological Association.

Hardeman, W., Johnston, M., Johnston, D. W., Bonetti, D., Wareham, N. J., & Kinmonth, A. L. (2002). Application of the theory of planned behaviour in behaviour change interventions: A systematic review. *Psychology and Health 17*(2), 125–158.

Hardy, M. A., & Quadagno, J. (1995). Satisfaction with early retirement: Making choices in the auto industry. *Journal of Gerontology: Social Sciences, 50B,* S217–S228.

Hare, J., Pratt, C., & Nelson, C. (1992). Agreement between patients and their self-selected surrogates on difficult medical decisions. *Archives of Internal Medicine, 52,* 1049–1054.

Harpole, L. H., Williams, J. W. Jr., Olsen, M. K., Stechuchak, K. M., Oddone, E., Callahan, C. M., et al. (2005). Improving depression outcomes in older adults with comorbid medical illness. *General Hospital Psychiatry, 27*(1), 4–12.

Hartman-Stein, P. E. (2006). The basics of building and managing a geropsychology practice. In S. H. Qualls & B. G. Knight (Eds.), *Psychotherapy for depression in older adults* (pp. 229–249). Hoboken, NJ: John Wiley.

Hartman-Stein, P. E., & Georgoulakis, J. M. (2007). How Medicare shapes behavioral health practice with older adults in the U.S.: Issues and recommendations for practitioners.

In D. Gallagher-Thompson, L. W. Thompson, & A. M. Steffen (Eds.), *Behavioral and cognitive therapies with older adults* (pp. 323–334). New York: Springer.

Harwood, D. G., Sultzer, D. L., & Wheatley, M. V. (2000). Impaired insight in Alzheimer disease: Association with cognitive deficits, psychiatric symptoms, and behavioral disturbances. *Neuropsychiatry, Neuropsychology, and Behavioral Neurology, 13*, 83–88.

Hasher, L., Stoltzfus, E. R., Zacks, R. T., & Rypma, B. (1991). Age and inhibition. *Journal of Experimental Psychology: Learning, Memory, and Cognition, 17*, 163–169.

Hasher, L., Zachs, R. T., & May, C. P. (1999). Inhibitory control, circadian arousal, and age. In D. Gopher & A. Koriat (Eds.), *Attention and performance XVII* (pp. 653–675). Cambridge, MA: MIT Press.

Hawkins, N. A., Ditto, P. H., Danks, J. H., & Smucker, W. D. (2005). Micromanaging death: Process preferences, values, and goals in end-of-life medical decision making. *The Gerontologist, 45*(1), 107–117.

Hayes, S. C., Nelson, R. O., & Jarrett, R. B. (1989). The applicability of treatment utility. *American Psychologist, 44*, 1242–1243.

Haynes, S. N. & O'Brien, W. H. (2000). Principles and practice of behavioral assessment. New York: Kluwer Academic.

Hedden, T., & Gabrieli, J. D. (2004). Insights into the ageing mind: A view from cognitive neuroscience. *Nature Review Neuroscience, 5*, 87–96.

Hedrick, S. C., Chaney, E. F., Felker, B., Liu, C., Hasenberg, N., Heagerty, P., et al. (2003). Effectiveness of collaborative care depression treatment in Veterans' Affairs primary care. *Journal of Internal Medicine, 18*, 9–16.

Hegel, M., & Arean, P. A. (2003). *Problem-solving treatment for primary care: A treatment manual for depression.* Lebanon, NH: Project IMPACT, Dartmouth College.

Hegel, M., Dietrich, A. J., Seville, J. L., & Jordan, C. B. (2004). Training residents in problem-solving treatment of depression: A pilot feasibility and impact study. *Family Medicine, 36*, 204–208.

Heinemann, G. D., Farrell, M. P., & Schmitt, M. H. (1994). Groupthink theory and research: Implications for decision making in geriatric health care teams. *Educational Gerontology, 20*(1), 71–85.

Heinemann, G. D., & Zeiss, A. M. (2002). *Team performance in health care: Assessment and development.* New York: Kluwer.

Herman, K. C., Tucker, C. M., Ferdinand, L. A., Mirsu-Pau, A., Hasan, N. T., & Beato, C. (2007). Culturally sensitive health care and counseling psychology: An overview. *Counseling Psychologist, 35*, 633–649.

Hester, D. M. (Ed.). (2007). *Ethics by committee: A textbook on consultation, organization, and education for hospital ethics committees:* Lanham, MD: Rowman & Littlefield.

Hibbard, J. H., Jewett, J. J., Engelmann, S., & Tusler, M. (1998). Can Medicare beneficiaries make informed choices? *Health Affairs, 17*, 181–193.

Hill, C. E., O'Grady, K. E., & Elkin, I. (1992). Applying the collaborative study psychotherapy rating scale to rate therapist adherence in cognitive-behavior therapy, interpersonal therapy, and clinical management. *Journal of Consulting and Clinical Psychology, 60*, 73–79.

Hill, R. D. & Mansour, E. (2008). The role of positive aging in addressing the mental health needs of older adults. In D. Gallagher-Thompson, A. M. Steffen, & L. W. Thompson

(Eds.), *Handbook of behavioral and cognitive therapies with older adults* (pp. 309-322). New York, Springer.

Hinrichsen, G. A. (2000). Knowledge of and interest in geropsychology among psychology trainees. *Professional Psychology: Research and Practice, 31,* 442–445.

Hinrichsen, G. A. (2006). Why multicultural issues matter for practitioners working with older adults. *Professional Psychology: Research and Practice, 37,* 29–35.

Hinrichsen, G. A., & Clougherty, K. F. (2006). *Interpersonal psychotherapy for depressed older adults.* Washington, DC: American Psychological Association.

Hinrichsen, G. A., & McMeniman, M. (2002). The impact of geropsychology training. *Professional Psychology: Research and Practice, 33,* 337–340.

Hinrichsen, G. A., Myers, D. S., & Stewart, D. (2000). Doctoral internship training opportunities in clinical geropsychology. *Professional Psychology: Research and Practice, 31,* 88–92.

Hinrichsen, G., Zeiss, A., Karel, M., Molinari, V. (2010). Competency-based training in doctoral internship and postdoctoral fellowships. *Training and Education in Professional Psychology, 4*(21), 91–98.

Hinrichsen, G. A., & Zweig, R. A. (2005). Models of training in clinical geropsychology. *Gerontology and Geriatrics Education, 25*(4), 1–4.

Holahan, C. J., Moos, R. H., Holahan, C. K., Brennan, P. L., & Schutte, K. K. (2005). Stress generation, avoidance coping, and depressive symptoms: A 10-year model. *Journal of Consulting and Clinical Psychology, 73,* 658–666.

Holstein, M. B., & Mitzen, P. B. (Eds.). (2001). *Ethics in community-based elder care.* New York: Springer.

Hornung, C. A., Eleazer, G. P., Strothers, H. S., III, Wieland, G. D., Eng, C., McCann, R., et al. (1998). Ethnicity and decision-makers in a group of frail older people. *Journal of the American Geriatrics Society, 46*(3), 280–286.

Horowitz, M., & Kaltreider, N. (1979). Brief therapy of the stress response syndrome. *Psychiatric Clinics of North America, 2,* 365–377.

Horvath, A. O., & Bedi, R. P. (2002). The alliance. In J. C. Norcross (Ed.), *Psychotherapy relationships that work: Therapist contributions and responsiveness to patient needs* (pp. 37–69). London: Oxford University Press.

Howarth, A., & Shone, G. R. (2006). Ageing and the auditory system. *Postgraduate Medical Journal, 82,* 166–171.

Hoyer, W. J., & Roodin, P. A. (2003). Adult development and aging (5th ed.). Boston, MA: McGraw-Hill.

Huber, R., Borders, K. W., Badrak, K., Netting, F. E., & Nelson, H. W. (2001). National standards for the long-term care ombudsman program and a tool to assess compliance: The Huber Badrak borders scales. *The Gerontologist, 41,* 264–271.

Hulicka, I. M., & Whitbourne, S. K. (1990). Teaching courses on the psychology of adult development and aging. In I. A. Parham, L. W. Poon, & I. C. Siegler (Eds.), *ACCESS: Aging curriculum content for education in the social-behavioral sciences* (pp. 1–37). New York: Springer.

Hunkeler, E. M., Katon, W., Tang, L., Williams, J. W. Jr., Kroenke, K., Lin, E. H., et al. (2006). Long term outcomes from the IMPACT randomised trial for depressed elderly patients in primary care. *British Medical Journal, 4,* 259–263.

Hussian, R. (1981). *Geriatric psychology: A behavioral perspective.* New York: Van Nostrand Reinhold.

Hussian, R. A. & Lawrence, P. S. (1981). Social reinforcement of activity and problem-solving training in the treatment of depressed institutionalized elderly patients. *Cognitive Therapy and Research, 5,* 57-69.

Hyer, L., & Intrieri, R. C. (2006). *Geropsychological interventions in long term care.* New York: Springer.

Hyer, L., Leventhal, G., & Gartenberg, M. (2005). Geropsychology: Integrated training at the intern level. *Gerontology and Geriatrics Education, 25,* 41–61.

Institute of Medicine. (2001). *Crossing the quality chasm: A new health system for the 21st century.* Washington, DC: National Academies Press.

Institute of Medicine. (2008). *Retooling for an aging America: Building the health care workforce.* Washington, DC: National Academies Press.

Institute of Medicine, Board of Health Sciences Policy, Committee on Understanding and Eliminating Racial and Ethnic Disparities in Health Care. (2002). *Unequal treatment: Confronting racial and ethnic disparities in health care.* Washington, DC: National Academy of Science.

Iwasaki, M., Tazeau, Y. N., Kimmel, D., Baker, N. L., & McCallum, T. J. (2009). Gerodiversity and social justice: Voices of minority elders. In J. L. Chin (Ed.), *Diversity in mind and action: Vol. 3. Social, psychological, and political challenges* (pp. 71–90). Westport, CT: Praeger.

Jackson, G. R., & Owsley, C. (2003). Visual dysfunction, neurodegenerative diseases, and aging. *Neurologic Clinics of North America, 21,* 709–728.

Jacobs, S. C., & Formati, M. J. (1998). Older adults and geriatrics. In S. Roth-Roemer, S. E. R. Kurpius, & C. Carmin (Eds.), *The emerging role of counseling psychology in health care* (pp. 309–329). New York: W.W. Norton.

Jeste, D. V., Alexopolous, G. S., Bartels, S. J., Cummings, J. L., Gallo, J. J., Gottlieb, G. L., et al. (1999). Consensus statement on the upcoming crisis in geriatric mental health. *Archives of General Psychiatry, 56,* 848–853.

Jeste, D. V., Blazer, D. G., & First, M. (2005). Aging-related diagnostic variations: Need for diagnostic criteria appropriate for elderly psychiatric patients. *Biological Psychiatry, 58,* 265–271.

Joint Committee on Interprofessional Relations between the American Speech-Language-Hearing Association and Division 40 (Clinical Neuropsychology) of the American Psychological Association. (2007. *Structure and function of an interdisciplinary team for persons with acquired brain injury.* Retrieved on December 1, 2008, from: http://forms.apa.org/about/division/asha-form/ASHA-Division40.pdf.

Jonsen, A. R., Siegler, M., & Winslade, W. J. (1998). *Clinical ethics* (4th ed.). New York: McGraw-Hill.

Kalimo, R., Taris, T. W., & Schaufeli, W. B. (2003). The effects of past and anticipated future downsizing on survivor well-being: An equity perspective. *Journal of Occupational Health Psychology, 8,* 91–109.

Kane, R. A., & Caplan, A. L. (1990). *Everyday ethics: Resolving dilemmas in nursing home life.* New York: Springer.

Karel, M. J. (2000). The assessment of values in medical decision making. *Journal of Aging Studies, 14*(4), 403–422.

Karel, M. J. (2007a). Culture and medical decision making. In S. H. Qualls & M. Smyer (Eds.), *Changes in decision-making capacity in older adults: Assessment and intervention* (pp. 145–174). Hoboken, NJ: John Wiley.

Karel, M. J. (2007b). The Pikes Peak Model for training in professional geropsychology: Defining and building competencies for geropsychology practice [PowerPoint slides]. Retrieved January 09, 2009 from http://www.appic.org/Conference2007/Downloads/Pikes%20Peak%20Model%20-%20APPIC07.ppt. .

Karel, M. J. (2008). Ethical issues. In E. Rosowsky, J. Casciani, & M. Arnold (Eds.), *Geropsychology and long term care: A practitioner's guide* (pp. 111–123). New York: Springer.

Karel, M. J., Emery, E. E., Molinari, V., & CoPGTP Task Force on the Assessment of Geropsychology Competencies. (in press). Development of a tool to evaluate geropsychology knowledge and skill competencies. *International Psychogeriatrics*.

Karel, M. J., & Gatz, M. (1996). Factors influencing life-sustaining treatment decisions in a community sample of families. *Psychology and Aging, 11*(2), 226–234.

Karel, M. J., & Hinrichsen, G. (2000). Treatment of depression in late life: Psychotherapeutic interventions. *Clinical Psychology Review, 20,* 707–729.

Karel, M. J., Knight, B. G., Duffy, M., Hinrichsen, G. A., & Zeiss, A. (2010). Attitude, knowledge, and skill competencies for practice in professional geropsychology: Implications for training and building a geropsychology workforce. *Training and Education in Professional Psychology, 4*(2), 75–84.

Karel, M. J., Molinari, V., Gallagher-Thompson, D., & Hillman, S. L. (1999). Postdoctoral training in professional geropsychology: A survey of fellowship graduates. *Professional Psychology: Research and Practice, 30,* 617–622.

Karel, M. J., & Moye, J. (2005). Geropsychology training in a VA nursing home setting. *Gerontology and Geriatrics Education, 25,* 83–107.

Karel, M. J., & Moye, J. (2006). The ethics of dementia caregiving. In S. Loboprabhu, V. Molinari & J. Lomax (Eds.), *Supporting the caregiver in dementia: A guide for health care professional* (pp. 261–284). Baltimore, MD: Johns Hopkins University Press.

Karel, M. J., Moye, J., Bank, A., & Azar, A. R. (2007). Three methods of assessing values for advance care planning: Comparing persons with and without dementia. *Journal of Aging and Health, 19*(1), 123–151.

Karel, M. J., Ogland-Hand, S. & Gatz, M. (2002). *Assessing and treating late-life depression.* New York: Basic Books.

Karel, M. J., Powell, J., & Cantor, M. D. (2004). Using a values discussion guide to facilitate communication in advance care planning. *Patient Education and Counseling, 55*(1), 22–31.

Karel, M. J., Qualls, S. H., & Smyer, M. A. (2007). Culture and medical decision making. In *Changes in decision-making capacity in older adults: Assessment and intervention* (pp. 145–174). Hoboken, NJ : John Wiley.

Karlawish, J. H., Kim, S. Y. H., Knopman, D., van Dyck, C. H., James, B. D., & Marson, D. (2008a). Interpreting the clinical significance of capacity scores for informed consent in Alzheimer disease clinical trials. *American Journal of Geriatric Psychiatry, 16*(7), 568–574.

Karlawish, J. H., Kim, S. Y. H., Knopman, D., van Dyck, C. H., James, B. D., & Marson, D. (2008b). The views of Alzheimer disease patients and their study partners on proxy consent for clinical trial enrollment. *American Journal of Geriatric Psychiatry, 16*(3), 240–247.

Karlawish, J. H., Quill, T., & Meier, D. (1999). A consensus-based approach to providing palliative care to patients who lack decision-making capacity. *Annals of Internal Medicine, 130*, 835–840.

Kaslow, N. J., Rubin, N. J., Bebeau, M. J., Leigh, I. W., Lichtenberg, J. W., Nelson, P. D., et al. (2007). Guiding principles and recommendations for the assessment of competence. *Professional Psychology: Research and Practice, 38*, 441–451.

Kastenbaum, R. (1963). The reluctant therapist. *Geriatrics, 18*, 296–301.

Kastenbaum, R., Barber, T. X., Wilson, S. C., Ryder, B. L., & Hathaway, L. B. (1981). *Old, sick and helpless: Where therapy begins.* Cambridge, MA: Ballinger.

Kaszniak, A. W. (1990). Psychological assessment of the aging individual. In J. E. Birren & K. W. Schaie (Eds.), *Handbook of the psychology of aging* (3rd ed., pp. 427–445). New York: Academic Press.

Katon, W. J. (2008). The comorbidity of diabetes mellitus and depression. *American Journal of Medicine, 121*, S8–S15.

Katon, W., Russo, J., Von Korff, M., Lin, E., Simon, G., Bush, T., et al. (2002). Long-term effects of a collaborative care intervention in persistently depressed primary care patients. *Journal of Geriatric Internal Medicine, 17*, 741–748.

Katzelnick, D. J., Kobak, K. A., Greist, J. H., Jefferson, J. W., & Henk, H. J. (1997). Effect of primary care treatment of depression on service use by patients with high medical expenditures. *Psychiatric Services, 48*, 59–64.

Katzelnick, D. J., Simon, G. E., Pearson, S. D., Manning, W. G., Helstad, C. P., Henk, H. J., et al. (2000). Randomized trial of a depression management program in high utilizers of medical care. *Archives of Family Medicine, 9*, 345–351.

Kiecolt-Glaser, J. K., & Glaser, R. (2002). Depression and immune function: Central pathways to morbidity and mortality. *Journal of Psychosomatic Research, 53*, 873–876.

Kim, S. Y., Appelbaum, P. S., Jeste, D. V., & Olin, J. T. (2004). Proxy and surrogate consent in geriatric neuropsychiatric research: Update and recommendations. *American Journal of Psychiatry, 161*, 797–806.

Kim, S. Y., Caine, E. D., Currier, G. W., Leibovici, A., & Ryan, J. M. (2001). Assessing the competence of persons with Alzheimer's disease in providing informed consent for participation in research. *American Journal of Psychiatry, 158*, 712–717.

Kimmel, D., Rose, T., & David, S. (Eds.). (2006). *Lesbian, gay, bisexual, and transgender aging: Research and clinical perspectives.* New York: Columbia University Press.

King, D. A., & Markus, H. E. (2000). Mood disorders in older adults. In S. K. Whitbourne (Ed.), *Psychopathology in later life* (pp. 141–172). New York: Wiley.

Kirsch, I., Jungeblut, A., Jenkins, L., & Kolstad, A. (1993). *Adult literacy in America: A first look at the results of the National Adult Literacy Survey.* Washington, DC: U.S. Department of Education, National Center for Education Statistics.

Kite, M. E., & Wagner, L. S. (2002). Attitudes toward older adults. In T. D. Nelson (Ed.), *Ageism: Stereotyping and prejudice against older persons* (pp. 129–161). Cambridge, MA: MIT Press.

Klapp, R., Tschantz, K., & Unützer, J. (2003). Caring for mental disorders in the United States: A focus on older adults. *Journal of the American Geriatrics Society, 11*, 517–524.

Klemmack, D. L., Roff, L. L., Parker, M. W., Koenig, H. G., Sawyer, P., & Allman, R. M. (2007). A cluster analysis typology of religiousness/spirituality among older adults. *Research on Aging, 29*, 163–183.

Knight, B. G. (1986). *Psychotherapy with older adults.* Newbury Park, CA: Sage.

Knight, B. G. (2004). *Psychotherapy with older adults (3rd ed.)*. Thousand Oaks, CA: Sage.

Knight, B. G., Karel, M. J., Hinrichsen, G. A., Qualls, S. H., & Duffy, M. (2009). Pikes Peak model for training in professional geropsychology. *American Psychologist,* 64(3), 205-214.

Knight, B. G. & Lee, L. O. (2008). Contextual adult lifespan theory for adapting psychotherapy. In K. Laidlaw & B. Knight (Eds.), *Handbook of emotional disorders in later life: Assessment and treatment* (pp. 59-88). New York, NY: Oxford.

Knight, B. G., Santos, J., Teri, L. & Lawton, M. P. (1995). The development of training in clinical geropsychology. In B. G. Knight, L. Teri, P. Wohlford & J. Santos (Eds) *Mental health services for older adults: Implications for training and practice.* American Psychological Association. Washington, DC: American Psychological Association.

Knight, B. G., Teri, L., Wohlford, P., & Santos, J. (Eds.). (1995). *Mental health services for older adults: Implications for training and practice in geropsychology.* Washington, DC: American Psychological Association.

Koder, D. A., & Helmes, E. (2008.) Predictors of working with older adults in an Australian psychologist sample: Revisiting the influence of contact. *Professional Psychology: Research and Practice, 39,* 276–282.

Kogan, J., & Edelstein, B. (2004). Modification and psychometric examination of a self-report measure of fear in older adults. *Journal of Anxiety Disorders, 18,* 397–409.

Koppelman, E. R. (2002). Dementia and dignity: Towards a new method of surrogate decision making. *Journal of Medicine and Philosophy, 27,* 65–85.

Koropeckyj-Cox, T. (2002). Beyond parental status: Psychological well-being in middle and old age. *Journal of Marriage and Family, 64,* 957–971.

Krahn, D. D., Bartels, S. J., Coakley, E., Oslin, D. W., Chen, H., McIntyre, J., et al. (2006). PRISM-E: Comparison of integrated care and enhanced specialty referral models in depression outcomes. *Psychiatric Services, 57*(7), 946–953.

Kramer, A. F., Boot, W. R., McCarley, J. S., Peterson, M. S., Colcombe, A., & Scialfa, C. T. (2006). Aging, memory and visual search. *Acta Psychologica, 122,* 288–304.

Krisberg, K. (2005). Cultural competencies needed to serve all older Americans. *Nation's Health, 35,* 1–30.

La Roche, M. J., & Maxie, A. (2003). Ten considerations in addressing cultural differences in psychotherapy. *Professional Psychology: Research and Practice, 34,* 180–186.

Laidlaw, K. & Thompson, L. W. (2008). Cognitive behaviour therapy with depressed older people. In K. Laidlaw & B. Knight (Eds.), *Handbook of emotional disorders in later life: Assessment and treatment* (pp. 91-116). New York, NY: Oxford.

Laidlaw, K., Thompson, L. W., Dick-Siskin, L., & Gallagher-Thompson, D. (2003). *Cognitive behaviour therapy with older people.* New York: Wiley.

Lamme, S., Dykstra, P. A., & Broese Van Groenou, M. I. (1996). Rebuilding the network: New relationships in widowhood. *Personal Relationships, 3,* 337–349.

Lau, A. S. (2006). Making the case for selective and directed cultural adaptations of evidence-based treatments: Examples from parent training. *Clinical Psychology: Science and Practice, 13,* 295–310.

Lawton, M. P. (1975). *Planning and managing housing for the elderly*. New York: John Wiley.

Lawton, M. P., & Nahemow, L. (1973). Ecology and the aging process. In C. Eisdorfer & M. P. Lawton (Eds.), *The psychology of adult development and aging* (pp. 619–674). Washington, D.C.: American Psychological Association.

Lazarus, L. W. (1980). Self psychology and psychotherapy with the elderly: Theory and practice. *Journal of Geriatric Psychiatry, 13*, 69–88.

Leichsenring, F., & Leibing, E. (2007). Psychodynamic psychotherapy: A systematic review of techniques, indications and empirical evidence. *Psychology and Psychotherapy: Theory, Research and Practice, 80*, 217–228.

Lemme, B. H. (2006). *Development in adulthood (4th Ed.)*. Boston, MA: Allyn & Bacon.

Lenze, E. J., Munin, M. C., Skidmore, E. R., Dew, M. A., Rogers, J. C., Whyte, E. M., et al. (2007). Onset of depression in elderly persons after hip fracture: Implications for prevention and early intervention of late-life depression. *Journal of the American Geriatrics Society, 55*, 81–86.

Lerner, R. M. (1984). *On the nature of human plasticity*. New York: Cambridge University Press.

Levant, R. F. (2008). The 2005 White House Conference on Aging: Psychology and the aging Boomers. *Psychological Services, 5*, 94–96.

Levy, B. R., Slade, M. D., Kunkel, S. R., & Kasl, S. V. (2002). Longevity increased by positive self-perceptions of aging. *Journal of Personality and Social Psychology, 83*, 261–270.

Levy, B., Zonderman, A., Slade, M., & Ferrucci, L. (2009, March). Age stereotypes held earlier in life predict cardiovascular events in later life. *Psychological Science, 20*, 296–298.

Lewinsohn, P. M., Teri, L., & Hautzinger, M. (1984) Training clinical psychologists for work with older adults: A working model. *Professional Psychology: Research and Practice, 15*, 187–202.

Lichstein, K. L. (2000). Relaxation. In K. L. Lichstein & C. M. Morin (Eds.), *Treatment of late-life insomnia* (pp. 185–206). Thousand Oaks, CA: Sage.

Lichstein, K. L. & Morin, C. M. (Eds.) (2000). *Treatment of late life insomnia*. Thousand Oaks, CA: Sage.

Lichstein, K. L., Reidel, B. W., Wilson, N. M., Lester, K. W., & Aguillard, R. N. (2001). Relaxation and sleep compression for late-life insomnia: A placebo-controlled trial. *Journal of Consulting and Clinical Psychology, 69*, 227–239.

Lichtenberg, P. (1999). *Handbook of assessment in clinical gerontology*. New York: John Wiley & Sons.

Lichtenberg, P. (in press). *Handbook of assessment in clinical gerontology (2nd Ed.)*. New York: John Wiley & Sons.

Lichtenberg, P. A., Smith, M., Frazer, D., Molinari, V., Rosowsky, E., Crose, R. et al. (1998). Standards for psychological services in long-term care facilities. *The Gerontologist, 38*(1), 122–127.

Lin, E. H. B. (2008). Depression and osteoarthritis. *American Journal of Medicine, 21*, S16–S19.

Lin, E. H. B., Katon, W., Von Korff, M., Tang, L., Williams, J. W. Jr., Kroenke, K., et al. (2003). Effect of improving depression care on pain and functional outcomes among older adults with arthritis: A randomized controlled trial. *JAMA, 290*(18), 2428–2434.

Lindstrom, T. C. (1995). Anxiety and adaptation in bereavement. *Anxiety, Stress and Coping: An International Journal, 8,* 251–261.

Liu, C. F., Cedrick, S. C., Chaney, E. F., Heagerty, P., Felker, B., Hasenberg, N., et al. (2003). Cost effectiveness of collaborative care for depression in a primary care veteran population. *Psychiatric Services, 54,* 698–704.

LoConto, D. G. (1998). Death and dreams: A sociological approach to grieving and identity. *Omega—Journal of Death and Dying, 37,* 171–185.

Lubin, B., Brady, K., Thomas, E. A., & Whitlock, R. V. (1986). Training in geropsychology at the doctoral level: 1984. *Journal of Clinical Psychology, 42,* 387–391.

Lucas, R. E., Clark, A. E., Georgellis, Y., & Diener, E. (2003). Reexamining adaptation and the set point model of happiness: Reactions to changes in marital status. *Journal of Personality and Social Psychology, 84,* 527–539.

Lupsakko, T., Mantyjarvi, M., Kautiainen, H., & Sulkava, R. (2002). Combined hearing and visual impairment and depression in a population aged 75 years and older. *International Journal of Geriatric Psychiatry, 17,* 808–813.

Lustman, P. J., & Clouse, R. E. (2005). Depression in diabetic patients: The relationship between mood and glycemic control. *Journal of Diabetes and Its Complications, 19,* 113–122.

Lyden, M. (2007). Assessment of sexual consent capacity. *Sexual Disabilities, 25,* 3–20.

Lyketsos, C. G., Kozauer, N., & Rabins, P. V. (2007). Psychiatric manifestations of neurologic disease: Where are we headed? *Dialogues in Clinical Neuroscience, 9,* 111–124.

Macdonald, C. J., Stodel, E. J., & Chambers, L. W. (2008). An online interprofessional learning resource for physicians, pharmacists, nurse practitioners, and nurses in long-term care: Benefits, barriers, and lessons learned. *Informatics for Health Social Care, 33*(1), 21–38.

Mackin, S. R., & Areán, P. A. (2005). Evidence-based psychotherapeutic interventions for geriatric depression. *Psychiatric Clinics of North America, 28,* 805–820.

Madden, D. J. (2001). Speed and timing of behavioural processes. In J. E. Birren & K. W. Schaie (Eds.), *Handbook of the psychology of aging* (5th ed., pp. 288–312). San Diego, CA: Academic Press.

Maeise, D. R. (2002). Healthy people 2010: Leading health indicators for women. *Women's Health Issues, 12,* 155–164.

Manly, J. J. (2006). Cultural issues. In D. K. Attix & K. A. Welsh-Bohmer (Eds.), *Geriatric neuropsychology: Assessment and intervention* (pp. 198–222). New York: Guilford.

Manly, J. J., Byrd, D. A., Touradji, P., & Stern, Y. (2004). Acculturation, reading level, and neuropsychological test performance among African American elders. *Applied Neuropsychology, 11*(1), 37–46.

Mann, J. (1973). *Time-limited psychotherapy.* Cambridge, MA: Harvard University Press.

Marsh, L. (2000). Anxiety disorders in Parkinson's disease. *International Review of Psychiatry, 12,* 307–318.

Marsh, L. (2008). Parkinson's disease. In C. G. Lyketsos, P. V., Rabins, J. R. Lipsey, & P. R. Slavney (Eds.), *Psychiatric aspects of neurologic disease: Practical approaches to patient care* (p.189). New York: Oxford University Press.

Marsh, L., McDonald, W. M., Cummings, J., & Ravina, B. (2005). Provisional diagnostic criteria for depression in Parkinson's disease: Report on NINDS/NIMH work group. *Movement Disorders, 21,* 148–158.

Marson, D. C. (2001). Loss of financial competency in dementia: Conceptual and empirical approaches. *Aging, Neuropsychology, and Cognition, 8*(3), 164–181.

Marson, D. C., & Hebert, K. (2005). Assessing civil competencies in older adults with dementia: Consent capacity, financial capacity, and testamentary capacity. In Larrabee (Ed.), *Forensic neuropsychology: A scientific approach* (pp. 334–377). New York: Oxford University Press.

Marson, D. C., & Huthwaite, J. S. (2005). An unexpected excursion: Sexual consent capacity in a nursing home patient with Alzheimer's disease. In R. L. Heilbronner (Ed.), *Forensic neuropsychology casebook* (pp. 146–164). New York: Guilford Press.

Marson, D. C., McInturff, B., Hawkins, L., Bartolucci, A., & Harrell, L. (1997). Consistency of physician judgments of capacity to consent in mild Alzheimer's disease. *Journal of the American Geriatrics Society, 45*(4), 453–457.

Marson, D. C., Sawrie, S., McInturff, B., Snyder, S., Chatterjee, A., Stalvey, T., et al. (2000). Assessing financial capacity in patients with Alzheimer's disease: A conceptual model and prototype instrument. *Archives of Neurology, 57,* 877–884.

Martens, A., Greenberg, J., Schimel, J., & Landau, M. J. (2004). Ageism and death: Effects of mortality salience and perceived similarity to elders on reactions to elderly people. *Personality and Social Psychology Bulletin, 30,* 1524–1536.

Massachusetts General Hospital Institute for Health Policy, the Disparities Solution Center. (2009). *Improving quality and achieving equity: A guide for hospital leaders.* Retrieved March 11, 2009, from www2.massgeneral.org/disparitiessolutions/guide.html.

Matthews, L., & Marwit, S. (2004, November). Complicated grief and the trend toward cognitive-behavioral therapy. *Death Studies, 28*(9), 849-863.

Mays, V. M. (2000). A social justice agenda. *American Psychologist, 55,* 326–327.

McCrae, R. R. (2002). The maturation of personality psychology: Adult personality development and psychological well-being. *Journal of Research in Personality, 36,* 307–317.

McCrae, R. R., & Costa, P. T. J. (2003). *Personality in adulthood: A five-factor theory perspective* (2nd ed.). New York: Guilford.

McCurry, S., Logsdon, R., Teri, L., & Vitiello, M. (2007, March). Evidence-based psychological treatments for insomnia in older adults. *Psychology and Aging, 22*(1), 18-27.

McQuaid, J. R., Granholm, E., McClure, F. S., Roepke, S., Pedrelli, P., Patterson, T. L., et al. (2000). Development of an integrated cognitive-behavioral and social skills training intervention for older patients with schizophrenia. *The Journal of Psychotherapy Practice and Research, 9,* 149-156.

Mehrotra, C. M., & Fried, S. B. (2002). Assessment of an online course on adult development, aging, and diversity. *Gerontology and Geriatrics Education, 23,* 49–57.

Mellor, M. J., & Brownell, P. J. (Eds.). (2006). *Elder abuse and mistreatment: Policy, practice, and research.* New York: Routledge.

Mezey, M. D., Cassel, C. D., Bottrell, M. M., Hyer, K., Howe, J. L., & Fulmer, T. T. (Eds.). (2002). *Ethical patient care: A casebook for geriatric health care teams.* Baltimore, MD: Johns Hopkins University Press.

Mezey, M., Teresi, J., Ramsey, G., Mitty, E., & Bobrowitz, T. (2000). Decision-making capacity to execute a heath care proxy: Development and testing of guidelines. *Journal of the American Geriatrics Society, 48*(2), 179–187.

Miller, M. D. (2009). *Clinician's guide to interpersonal psychotherapy in late life: Helping cognitively impaired or depressed elders and their caregivers.* New York: Oxford University Press.

Mischel, W. (1968). *Personality and assessment.* New York: Wiley.

Molinari, V., Karel, M., Jones, S., Zeiss, A., Cooley, S. G., Wray, L., et al. (2003). Recommendations about the knowledge and skills required of psychologists working with older adults. *Professional Psychology: Research and Practice, 34,* 435–443.

Molinari, V., McCullough, L., Workman, R., & Coverdale, J. (2004). Geriatric assent. *Journal of Clinical Ethics, 15,* 261–268.

Moore, K. M., & Georgoulakis, J. M. (2008, August). *Medicare participation, billing and fraud's red flags.* Presentation at the annual meeting of the American Psychological Association, Boston, MA.

Morin, C. M., Colecchi, C., Stone, J., Sood, R., & Brink, D. (1999). Behavioral and pharmacological therapies for late-life insomnia: A randomized controlled trial. *JAMA, 281,* 991–999.

Morin, C. M. & Epsie, C. A. (2003). *Insomnia: A clinical guide to assessment and treatment.* New York: Plenum.

Morley, S., Eccleston, C., & Williams, A. (1999). Systematic review and meta-analysis of randomized controlled trials of cognitive behaviour therapy and behaviour therapy for chronic pain in adults, excluding headache. *Pain, 80,* 1-13.

Moss, K. S. & Scogin, F. R. (2008). Behavioral and cognitive treatments for geriatric depression: An evidenced-based perspective. In D. Gallagher-Thompson, A.M. Steffen, & L. W. Thompson (Eds.), *Handbook of behavioral and cognitive therapies with older adults* (pp. 1-17). New York, NY: Springer.

Mossey, J. M., Knott, K. A., Higgins, M., & Talerico, K. (1996). Effectiveness of a psychosocial intervention, interpersonal counseling, for subdysthymic depression in medically ill elderly. *Journal of Gerontology: Medical Sciences, 51A,* M172– M178.

Moye, J. (2007). Clinical frameworks for capacity assessment. In S. H. Qualls & M. A. Smyer (Eds.), *Changes in decision-making capacity in older adults: Assessment and intervention* (pp. 177–190). Hoboken, NJ: John Wiley.

Moye, J., & Braun, M. (2007). Assessment of medical consent capacity and independent living. In S. H. Qualls & M. A. Smyer (Eds.), *Changes in decision-making capacity in older adults: Assessment and intervention* (pp. 205–236). Hoboken, NJ: John Wiley.

Moye, J., Butz, S. W., Marson, D. C., & Wood, E. (2007). A conceptual model and assessment template for capacity evaluation in adult guardianship. *The Gerontologist, 47*(5), 591–603.

Moye, J., Gurrera, R. J., Karel, M. J., Edelstein, B., & O'Connell, C. (2006). Empirical advances in the assessment of the capacity to consent to medical treatment: Clinical implications and research needs. *Clinical Psychology Review, 26*(8), 1054–1077.

Moye, J., & Marson, D. C. (2007). Assessment of decision-making capacity in older adults: An emerging area of practice and research. *Journal of Gerontology: Psychological Sciences and Social Sciences, 62B,* 3–11.

Moye, J., Wood, E., Edelstein, B., Wood, S., Bower, E. H., Harrison, J. A., et al. (2007). Statutory reform is associated with improved court practice: Results of a tri-state comparison. *Behavioral Sciences and the Law, 25*(3), 425–436.

Mueller, P. S., Hook, C. C., & Fleming, K. C. (2004). Ethical issues in geriatrics: A guide for clinicians. *Mayo Clinic Proceedings, 79*, 554–562.

Myers, J. E., & Schwiebert, V. L. (1996). *Competencies in gerontological counseling*. Alexandria, VA: American Counseling Association.

Myers, W.A. (1984). *Dynamic therapy of the older patient*. New York: Aronson.

Nasreddine, Z. S., Phillips, N. A., Bédirian, V., Charbonneau, S., Whitehead, V., Collin, I., et al. (2005). The Montreal Cognitive Assessment (MoCA): A brief screening tool for mild cognitive impairment. *Journal of the American Geriatrics Society, 53*, 695–699.

National Council for Community Behavioral Healthcare. (2006). Behavioral health/primary care integration: Finance, policy and integration of services. Retrieved December 8, 2008, from www.nccbh.org/who/industry/Primary%20Care%20Integration/Mauer_ Financing7-7- 06.pdf.

National Quality Forum. (2006, December). *A national framework and preferred practices for palliative and hospice care quality* (pp. 1–71). Washington, DC: National Quality Forum.

National Register of Health Service Providers in Psychology. (2009). Retrieved May 18, 2009 from http://www.nationalregister.org/.

Nelson, E. A., & Dannefer, D. (1992). Aged heterogeneity: Fact or fiction? The fate of diversity in gerontological research. *The Gerontologist, 32*, 17–23.

Nelson, H. W., Allen, P. D., & Cox, D. (2005). Rights-based advocacy in long-term care: Geriatric nursing and long term-care ombudsmen. *Clinical Gerontologist, 28*(4), 1–16.

Nelson-Becker, H., & Nakashima, M. (2007). Spiritual assessment in aging: A framework for clinicians. *Journal of Gerontological Social Work, 48*, 331–347.

Neugarten, B. (1973). Personality change in late life: A developmental perspective. *The psychology of adult development and aging* (pp. 311–335). Washington, DC: American Psychological Association.

Newton, N. A., & Jacobowitz, J. (1999). Transferential and countertransferential processes in therapy with older adults. In M. Duffy (Ed.), *Handbook of counseling and psychotherapy with older adults* (pp. 21–38). New York: Wiley.

Nezu, A. M. (2004). Problem solving and behavior therapy revisited. *Behavior Therapy, 35*, 1–33.

Nezu, A. M. (2005). Beyond cultural competence: Human diversity and the appositeness of assertive goals. *Clinical Psychology: Science and Practice, 12*, 19–24.

Nezu, A. M., Nezu, C. M., & Perri, M. G. (1989). *Problem-solving therapy for depression: Theory, research, and clinical guidelines*. Oxford: Wiley.

Niederehe, G., Gatz, M., Taylor, G. P., & Teri, L. (1995). The case for certification in clinical geropsychology and a framework for implementation. In B. G. Knight, L. Teri, P. Wohlford, & J. Santos (Eds.), *Mental health services for older adults* (pp.143–151). Washington, DC: American Psychological Association.

Nordhus, I. H., Nielsen, G. H., & Kvale, G. (1998). Psychotherapy with older adults. In I. H. Nordhus, G. R., VandenBos, & S. Berg (Eds.), *Clinical geropsychology* (pp. 289–311). Washington, DC: American Psychological Association.

Norman, S., Ishler, K., Ashcraft, L., & Patterson, M. (2000). Continuing education needs in clinical geropsychology: The practitioner's perspective. *Clinical Gerontologist, 22*(3/4), 37–50.

Norris, M. P. (2002). Psychologists' multiple roles in long-term care: Untangling confidentiality quandaries. *Clinical Gerontologist, 25*(3), 261–275.

Norris, M. P., Arnau, R. C., Bramson, R., & Meagher, M. W. (2004). The efficacy of somatic symptoms in assessing depression in older primary care patients. *Clinical Gerontologist, 27,* 43–57.

Norris, M., Molinari, V., & Rosowsky, E. (1998). Providing mental health care to older adults: Unraveling the maze of Medicare and managed care. *Psychotherapy, 35,* 490–497.

Norris, S. L., Engelgau, M. M., & Narayan, K. M. (2001). Effectiveness of self management training in type 2 diabetes: A systematic review of randomized, controlled trials. *Diabetes Care, 24,* 561–587.

Ogland-Hand, S. M. & Zeiss, A. M. (2000). In V. Molinari (Ed.), *Professional psychology in long term care* (pp. 257–277). New York: Hatherleigh Press.

Ong, A. D., Bergeman, C. S., Bisconti, T. L., & Wallace, K. A. (2006). Psychological resilience, positive emotions, and successful adaptation to stress in later life. *Journal of Personality and Social Psychology, 91,* 730–749.

Onrust, S. A., & Cuijpers, P. (2006). Mood and anxiety disorders in widowhood: A systematic review. *Aging and Mental Health, 10,* 327–334.

Oslin, D. W., Datto, C. J., Kallan, M. J., Katz, I. R., Edell, W. S., & TenHave, T. (2002). Association between medical comorbidity and treatment outcomes in late-life depression. *Journal of the American Geriatrics Society, 50,* 823–828.

Ott, C. H., & Lueger, R. J. (2002). Patterns of change in mental health status during the first two years of spousal bereavement. *Death Studies, 26,* 387–411.

Palmer, K., Berger, A. K., Monastero, R., Winblad, B., Backman, L., & Fratiglioni, L. (2007). Predictors of progression from mild cognitive impairment to Alzheimer disease. *Neurology, 68,* 1596–1602.

Park, C. L. (2007). Religious and spiritual issues in health and aging. In C. M. Aldwin, C. L. Park, & A. Spiro (Eds.), *Handbook of health psychology and aging* (pp. 313–337). New York: Guilford Press.

Parker, G. (2000). Classifying depression: Should paradigms lost be regained? *American Journal of Psychiatry, 157,* 1195–1203.

Parker, G., Roy, K., Hadzl-Pavlovic, D., Wilhelm, K., & Mitchell, P. (2001). The differential impact of age on the phenomenology of melancholia. *Psychological Medicine, 31,* 1231–1236.

Partners in Care Foundation. (2008). *Geriatric social work education (GSWEC): Advancing geriatric social work education.* Retrieved February 19, 2008, fromwww.picf.org/landing_pages/32,3.html.

Pearlman, R. A., Starks, H., Cain, K. C., & Cole, W. G. (2005). Improvements in advance care planning in the veterans affairs system: Results of a multifaceted intervention. *Archives of Internal Medicine, 165,* 667–674.

Pearlman, R., Starks, H., Cain, K., Rosengreen, D., & Patrick, D. (1998). *Your life, your choice—planning for future medical decisions: How to prepare a personalized living will* (No. PB#98159437). Springfield, VA: U.S. Department of Commerce, National Technical Information Service.

Pedrotti, J. T., Edwards, L. M., & Lopez, S. J. (2008). Working with multiracial clients in therapy: Bridging theory and practice. *Professional Psychology: Research and Practice, 39,* 192–201.

Persson, G. R., Persson, R. E., MacEntee, C. I., Wyatt, C. C., Hollender, L. G., & Kiyak, H. A. (2003). Periodontitis and perceived risk for periodontitis in elders with evidence of depression. *Journal of Clinical Periodontology, 30*, 691–696.

Persson, J., Nyberg, L., Lind, J., Larsson, A., Nilsson, L. G., Ingvar, M., & Buckner, R. L. (2006). Structure-function correlates of cognitive decline in aging. *Cerebral Cortex, 16*, 907–915.

Peters, R. (2006). Ageing and the brain. *Postgraduate Medical Journal, 82*, 84–88.

Pew Hispanic Center. (2004). *Assimilation and language. Pew Hispanic Center: Survey Brief.* Retrieved November 3, 2008, from http://pewhispanic.org/fies/factsheets/11.pdf.

Pichora-Fuller, M. K., & Souza, P. E. (2003). Effects of aging on auditory processing of speech. *International Journal of Audiology, 42*, S11–S16.

Plaut, V. C., Markus, H. R., & Lachman, M. E. (2003). Place matters: Consensual features and regional variation in American well-being and self. *Journal of Personality and Social Psychology, 83*, 160–184.

Playford, E. D., Dawson, L., Limbert, V., Smith, M., Ward, C. D., & Wells, R. (2000). Goal-setting in rehabilitation: Report of a workshop to explore professionals' perceptions of goal-setting. *Clinical Rehabilitation, 14*, 491–496.

Poon, L. (Ed.). (1980). *Aging in the 1980's.* Washington, DC: American Psychological Association.

Pope, K. S., & Vasquez, M. J. T. (2005). *How to survive and thrive as a therapist: Information, ideas and resources for psychologists in practice.* Washington, DC: American Psychological Association.

Prendergast, T. J. (2001). Advance care planning: Pitfalls, progress, promise. *Critical Care Medicine, 29*, N34–N39.

President's Commission for the Study of Ethical Problems in Medicine and Biomedical and Behavioral Research. (1983). *Deciding to forego life-sustaining treatment: A report on ethical, medical, and legal issues in treatment decisions.* Washington, DC: Government Printing Office.

Puchalski, C. M., Zhong, Z., Jacobs, M. M., Fox, E., Lynn, J., Harrold, J., et al. (2000). Patients who want their family and physician to make resuscitation decisions for them: Observations from support and help. *Journal of the American Geriatrics Society, 48*(5), S84–90.

Pulkki-Raback, L., Elovainio, M., Kivimaki, M., Raitakari, O. T., & Keltikangas-Jarvinen, L. (2005). Temperament in childhood predicts body mass in adulthood: The Cardiovascular Risk in Young Finns Study. *Health Psychology, 24*, 307–315.

Qualls, S. H. (1998). Training in geropsychology: Preparing to meet the demand. *Professional Psychology: Research and Practice, 29*, 23–28.

Qualls, S. H. (1999). Realizing power in intergenerational family hierarchies: Family reorganization when older adults decline. In M. Duffy (Ed.), *Handbook of counseling and psychotherapy with older adults* (pp. 228–241). Hoboken, NJ : John Wiley & Sons Inc.

Qualls, S. H., & Abeles, N. (2000). *Psychology and the aging revolution: How we adapt to a longer life.* Washington, DC: APA Press.

Qualls, S. H., & Czirr, R. (1988). Geriatric health teams: Classifying models of professional and team functioning. *The Gerontologist, 28*, 372–376.

Qualls, S., Duffy, M., & Crose, R. (1995). Supervision in community practicum settings. In B. G. Knight, L. Teri, P. Wohlford, & J. Santos (Eds.), *Mental health services for older adults: Implications for training and practice in geropsychology* (pp. 119-127). Washington, DC: American Psychological Association.

Qualls, S. H., & Knight, B. G. (2006). *Psychotherapy for depression in older adults*. Hoboken, NJ: John Wiley.

Qualls, S. H., Segal, D. L., Benight, C. C., & Kenny, M. P. (2005). Geropsychology training in a specialist geropsychology doctoral program. *Gerontology and Geriatrics Education, 25,* 21–40.

Qualls, S. H., Segal, D. L., Norman, S., Niederehe, G., & Gallagher-Thompson, D. (2002). Psychologists in practice with older adults: Current patterns, sources of training, and need for continuing education. *Professional Psychology: Research and Practice, 33*(5), 435–442.

Qualls, S. H., & Smyer, M. A. (2007). *Changes in decision-making capacity in older adults: Assessment and intervention*. Hoboken, NJ : John Wiley.

Quijano, L. M., Stanley, M. A., Petersen, N. J., Casado, B. L., Steinberg, E. H., Cully, J. A., et al. (2007). Healthy IDEAS: A depression intervention delivered by community-based case managers serving older adults. *Journal of Applied Gerontology, 26,* 139–156.

Ramírez, R. R., & de la Cruz, G. P. (2003). *Current population reports: The Hispanic population in the United States: March 2002* (U.S. Bureau of the Census, pp. 20–545). Washington, DC: U.S. Government Printing Office.

Raz, N., & Rodrigue, K. M. (2006). Differential aging of the brain: Patterns, cognitive correlates and modifiers. *Neuroscience and Biobehavioral Reviews, 30,* 730–748.

Reese, D. J., Melton, E., & Ciaravino, K. (2004). Programmatic barriers to providing culturally competent end-of-life care. *American Journal of Hospice and Palliative Medicine, 21,* 357–364.

Reid, M. C., Otis, J., Barry, L. C., & Kerns, R. D. (2003). Cognitive-behavioral therapy for chronic back pain in older persons: A preliminary study. *Pain Medicine, 4,* 223–230.

Reyes-Ortiz, C. A., Palaez, M., Koenig, H. G., & Mulligan, T. (2007). Religiosity and self-rated health among Latin American and Caribbean elders. *International Journal of Psychiatry in Medicine, 37,* 425–443.

Reynolds, C. F., III, Dew, M. A., Pollock, B. G., Mulsant, B. H., Frank, E., Miller, M. D., et al. (2006). Maintenance treatment of major depression in old age. *New England Journal of Medicine, 354,* 1130–1138.

Reynolds, C.F., III, Frank., E., Perel, J. M., Imber, S. D., Cornes, C., Miller, M. D., et al., (1999). Nortriptyline and interpersonal psychotherapy as maintenance therapies for recurrent major depression: A randomized controlled trial in patients older than 59 years. *JAMA, 281,* 39–45.

Riemsma, R. P., Kirwan, J. R., Taal, E., & Rasker, J. J. (2003). Patient education for adults with rheumatoid arthritis. *Cochrane Database of Systematic Reviews, 2*:CD003688.

Robb, C., Haley, W., Becker, M., Polivka, L., & Chwa, H. (2003). Attitudes towards mental health care in younger and older adults: Similarities and differences. *Aging and Mental Health, 7,* 142–152.

Robins, L. R., & Regier, D. A. (1991). *Psychiatric disorders in America*. New York: Free Press.

Rodolfa, E., Bent, R., Eisman, E., Nelson, P., Rehm, L., & Ritchie, P. (2005). A cube model for competency development: Implications for psychology educators and regulators. *Professional Psychology: Research and Practice, 36*(4), 347–354.

Rolita, L., & Freedman, M. (2008). Over-the-counter medication use in older adults. *Journal of Gerontological Nursing, 34,* 8–17.

Roper, B. L., Bieliauskas, L. A., & Peterson, M. R. (1996). Validity of the Mini-Mental State Examination and the Neurobehavioral Cognitive Status Examination in cognitive screening. *Neuropsychiatry, Neuropsychology and Behavioral Neurology, 9,* 54–57.

Rosenfeld, K. E., Wenger, N. S., & Kagawa-Singer, M. (2000). End-of-life decision making: A qualitative study of elderly individuals. *Journal of General Internal Medicine, 15,* 620–625.

Rothblum, E. D., Sholomskas, A. J., Berry, C., & Prusoff, B. A. (1982). Issues in clinical trials with the depressed elderly. *Journal of the American Geriatrics Society, 30,* 694–699.

Roy-Byrne, P. B., Katon, W., Cowley, D. S., & Russo, J. (2001). A randomized effectiveness trial of collaborative care for patients with panic disorder in primary care. *Archives of General Psychiatry, 58,* 869–876.

Rupp, D. E., Vodanovich, S. J., & Crede, M. (2006). Age bias in the workplace: The impact of ageism and causal attributions. *Journal of Applied Social Psychology, 36,* 1337–1364.

Rutman, D., & Silberfeld, M. (1992). A preliminary report on the discrepancy between clinical and test evaluations of competency. *Canadian Journal of Psychiatry, 37,* 634–639.

Sachs, G. A., Shega, J. W., & Cox-Hayley, D. (2004). Barriers to excellent end-of-life care for patients with dementia. *Journal of General Internal Medicine, 19,* 1057–1063.

Sackett, D. L., Rosenberg, W. M. C., Muir Gray, J. A., Haynes, R. B., & Richardson, W. S. (1996). Evidence based medicine: What it is and what it isn't. *British Medical Journal, 312,* 71.

Salthouse, T. (2004). What and when of cognitive aging. *Current Directions in Psychological Science, 13,* 140–144.

Salthouse, T. A., Hancock, H. E., Meinz, E. J., & Habrick, D. Z. (1996). Interrelations of age, visual acuity, and cognitive functioning. *Journal of Gerontology: Psychological Sciences and Social Sciences, 51B,* 317–330.

Salzman, C. (Ed.). (2005). *Clinical geriatric psychopharmacology* (4th ed.). New York: Lipincott Williams and Wilkins.

Santos, J. F., & VandenBos, G. R. (Eds.). (1982). *Psychology and the older adult: Challenges for training in the 1980's.* Washington, DC: American Psychological Association.

Saravay, S. M. (1996). Psychiatric interventions in the medically ill: Outcome and effectiveness research. *Psychiatric Clinics of North America, 19*(3), 467–480.

Schaie, K. W. (1983). What can we learn from the longitudinal study of adult psychological development? In K. W. Schaie (Ed.), *Longitudinal studies of adult psychological development* (pp. 1–19). New York: Guilford.

Schaie, K. W. (2008). A lifespan developmental perspective of psychological aging. In K. Laidlaw & B. Knight (Eds.), *Handbook of emotional disorders in later life: Assessment and treatment* (pp. 3–32). New York: Oxford.

Schaie, K. W., & Zanjani, F. (2006). Intellectual development across adulthood. In C. Hoare (Ed.), *Oxford handbook of adult development and learning* (pp. 99–122). New York: Oxford University Press.

Schiltz, K., Szentkuti, A., Guderian, S., Kaufmann, J., Munte, T. F., Heinze, H. J., et al. (2006). Relationship between hippocampal structure and memory function in elderly humans. *Journal of Cognitive Neuroscience, 18,* 990–1003.

Schim, S. M., Doorenbos, A. Z., & Borse, N. N. (2006). Enhancing cultural competence among hospice staff. *American Journal of Hospice and Palliative Medicine, 23*, 404–411.

Schuknecht, H. F., & Gacek, M. R. (1993). Cochlear pathology in presbyacusis. *Annals of Otology, Rhinology, and Laryngology, 102*, 1–16.

Schulz, R., Burgio, L., Burns, R., Eisdorfer, C., Gallagher-Thompson, D., Gitlin, L. N., et al. (2003). Resources for Enhancing Alzheimer's Caregiver Health (REACH): Overview, site-specific outcomes, and future directions. *The Gerontologist, 43*(4), 514–520.

Schulz, R., Mendelsohn, A., Haley, W., Mahoney, D., Allen, R., Zhang, S., et al. (2003). End-of-life care and the effects of bereavement on family caregivers of persons with dementia. *New England Journal of Medicine, 349*(20), 1936–1942.

Scogin, F. (2007). Introduction to the special section on evidence-based psychological treatments for older adults. *Psychology and Aging, 22*(1), 1–3.

Scogin, F., & McElreath, I. (1994). Efficacy of psychosocial treatments for geriatric depression: A quantitative review. *Journal of Consulting and Clinical Psychology, 57*, 403–407.

Scogin, F., Welsh, D., Hanson, A., Stump, J., & Coates, A. (2005). Evidence-based psychotherapies for depression in older adults. *Clinical Psychology: Sciences and Practice, 12*, 222–237.

Sechrest, L. (1963). Incremental validity: A recommendation. *Educational and Psychological Measurement, 23*, 153–158.

Segal, D. L., Qualls, S. H., & Smyer, M. A. (in press). *Aging and mental health (2nd Ed.).* Hoboken, NJ: Wiley.

Shear, M., Frank, E., Foa, E., Cherry, C., Reynolds, C., Vander Bilt, J., et al. (2001). Traumatic grief treatment: A pilot study. *American Journal of Psychiatry, 158*(9), 1506–1508.

Shear, K., Frank, E., Houck, P., & Reynolds, C. (2005). Treatment of complicated grief: A randomized controlled trial. *JAMA, 293*(21), 2601–2608.

Siegler, I. C., Costa, P. T., Brummett, B. H., Helms, M. J., Barefoot, J. C., Williams, R. B., et al. (2003). Patterns of change in hostility from college to midlife in the UNC Alumni Heart Study predict high-risk status. *Psychosomatic Medicine, 65*, 738–745.

Siegler, I. C., Gentry, W. D., & Edwards, C. D. (1979). Training in geropsychology: A survey of graduate and internship training programs. *Professional Psychology, 10*, 390–395.

Simon, G. E., Goldberg, D., Tiemens, B. G., & Ustun, T. B. (1999). Outcomes of recognized and unrecognized depression in an international primary care study. *General Hospital Psychiatry, 21*(2), 97–105.

Skarupski, K. A., Mendes de Leon, C. F., Bienias, J. L., Barnes, L. L., Everson-Rose, S. A., Wilson, R. S., et al. (2005). Black-white differences in depressive symptoms among older adults over time. *Journal of Gerontology: Psychological Sciences and Social Sciences, 60B*, 136–142.

Skultety, K. M., & Whitbourne, S. K. (2004). Gender differences in identity processes and self-esteem in middle and later adulthood. *Journal of Women and Aging, 16*, 175–188.

Skultety, K. M., & Zeiss, A. (2006). The treatment of depression in older adults in the primary care setting: An evidence based review. *Health Psychology, 25*, 665–674.

Sloane, R. B., Staples, F. R., & Schneider, L. S. (1985). Interpersonal psychotherapy versus nortriptyline for depression in the elderly. In G. Burrows, T. R. Norman, & L. Dennerstein (Eds.), *Clinical and pharmacological studies in psychiatric disorders* (pp. 344–346). London: John Libbey.

Smith, G. S., Gunning-Dixon, F. M., Lotrich, F. E., Taylor, W. D., & Evans, J. D. (2007). Translational research in late-life mood disorders: Implications for future intervention and prevention research. *Neuropsychopharmacology, 32*, 1857–1875.

Smits, S. J., Falconer, J. A., Herrin, J., Bowen, S. E., & Strasser, D. C. (2003). Patient-focused rehabilitation team cohesiveness in veterans administration hospitals. *Archives of Physical Medicine and Rehabilitation, 84*(9), 1332–1338.

Smyer, M., & Qualls, S.(1999). *Aging and mental health*. Malden, MA: Blackwell.

Sneed, J. R., Kasen, S., & Cohen, P. (2006). Early-life risk factors for late-onset depression. *International Journal of Geriatric Psychiatry, 22,* 663–667.

Sneed, J. R., & Whitbourne, S. K. (2003). Identity processing and self-consciousness in middle and later adulthood. *Journal of Gerontology: Psychological Sciences, 58B,* 313–319.

Sommers, L. S., Marton, K. I., Barbaccia, J. C., & Randolph, J. (2000). Physician, nurse, and social worker collaboration in primary care for chronically ill seniors. *Archives of Internal Medicine, 160,* 1825–1833.

Son, J., Erno, A., Shea, D. G., Femia, E. E., Zarit, S. H., & Stephens, M. A. P. (2007). The caregiver stress process and health outcomes. *Journal of Aging and Health, 19*(6), 871–887.

Speer, D. C., & Schneider, M. G. (2003). Mental health needs of older adults and primary care: Opportunity for interdisciplinary geriatric team practice. *Clinical Psychology: Science and Practice, 21,* 85–101.

Spiegel, J. P. (1965). Some cultural aspects of transference and countertransference. In M. N. Zald (Ed.), Social welfare institutions: A sociological reader (pp. 575–594). New York: John Wiley.

Stanely, M. A., & Beck, J. G. (2000). Anxiety disorders. *Clinical Psychology Review, 20,* 731–754.

Steffen, A. M, Gant, J. R., & Gallagher-Thompson, D. (2008). Reducing psychosocial distress in family caregivers. In D. Gallagher-Thompson, A. M. Steffen, & L. W. Thompson (Eds.), *Handbook of behavioral and cognitive therapies with older adults* (pp. 102–117). New York: Springer.

Stern, P. C., Carstensen, L. L., & The Committee on Future Directions for Cognitive Research on Aging (2000). *The aging mind: Opportunities in aging research.* Washington DC: National Academies Press.

Steuer, J. L., Mintz, J., Hammen, C. L., Hill, M. A., Jarvik, L. F., McCarley, T., et al. (1984). Cognitive-behavioral and psychodynamic group psychotherapy in treatment of geriatric depression. *Journal of Consulting and Clinical Psychology, 52,* 180–189.

Stoehr, G. P., Ganguli, M., Seaberg, E. C., Echement, D. A., & Belle, S. Over-the-counter medication use in an older rural community: The MOVIES Project. *Journal of the American Geriatrics Society, 45,* 158–165.

Stone, A. C., & Nici, L. (2007). Other systemic manifestations of chronic obstructive pulmonary disease. *Clinical Chest Medicine, 28,* 553–557.

Storandt, M. (1983). Understanding senile dementia: A challenge for the future, *International Journal of Aging and Human Development, 16*(1), 1–6.

Storandt, M., Siegler, I. C., & Elias, M. F. (Eds.). (1978). *The clinical psychology of aging.* New York: Plenum Press

Strasser, D. C., Falconer, J. A., Stevens, A. B., Uomoto, J. M., Herrin, J., Bowen, S. E., et al. (2008). Team training and stroke rehabilitation outcomes: A cluster randomized trial. *Archives of Physical Medicine and Rehabilitation, 89*(1), 10–15.

Strasser, D. C., Uomoto, J. M., & Smits, S. J. (2008). The interdisciplinary team and polytrauma rehabilitation: Prescription for partnership. *Archives of Physical Medicine and Rehabilitation, 89*(1), 179–181.

Strauss, E., Spreen, O., & Hunter, M. (2000). Implications of test revisions for research. *Psychological Assessment, 12,* 237–244.

Stroebe, M. (2001). Gender differences in adjustment to bereavement: An empirical and theoretical review. *Review of General Psychology, 5,* 62–83.

Stroebe, M., & Schut, H. (1999). The dual process model of coping with bereavement: Rationale and description. *Death Studies, 23*(3), 197–224.

Stuart, R. B. (2004). Twelve practical suggestions for achieving multicultural competence. *Professional Psychology: Research and Practice, 35,* 3–9.

Subramaniam, H., Dennis, M. S., & Byrne, E. J. (2006). The role of vascular risk factors in late onset bipolar disorder. *International Journal of Geriatric Psychiatry, 22,* 733–737.

Substance Abuse and Mental Health Services Administration. (2005). *SAMHSAiIssues consensus statement on mental health recovery.* Retrieved November 27, 2008, from www.samhsa.gov/news/newsreleases/060215_consumer.htm.

Sue, D. W. (2008). Multicultural organizational consultation: A social justice perspective. *Counseling Psychology Journal: Practice and Research, 60,* 157–169.

Sue, D. W., Arredondo, P., & McDavis, R. J. (1992). Multicultural counseling competencies: A call to the profession. *Journal of Counseling and Development, 70,* 477–486.

Sue, D. W., & Sue, D. (2008). *Counseling the culturally diverse: Theory and practice.* Hoboken, NJ: John Wiley.

Suhl, J., Simons, P., Reedy, T., & Garrick, T. (1994). Myth of substituted judgment: Surrogate decision making regarding life support is unreliable. *Archives of Internal Medicine, 154,* 90–96.

Sullivan, H. S. (1953). *The interpersonal theory of psychiatry.* New York: Norton.

Tariq, S. H., Tumosa, M., Chibnall, J. T., Perry H. M., III, & Morley, J. E. (2006). Comparison of the Saint Louis University mental status examination and the mini-mental state examination for detecting dementia and mild neurocognitive disorder-a pilot study. *American Journal of Geriatric Psychiatry, 14*(11), 900–910.

Taylor, R. J., Chatters, L. M., & Jackson, J. S. (2007). Religious and spiritual involvement among older African Americans, Caribbean blacks, and non-Hispanic whites: Findings from the national survey of American life. *Journal of Gerontology: Psychological Sciences and Social Sciences, 62B,* S238–S250.

Teno, J. M., Licks, S., Lynn, J., Wenger, N., Connors, A. F., Phillips, R. S., et al. (1997). Do advance directives provide instructions that direct care? *Journal of the American Geriatrics Society, 45*(4), 508–512.

Teri L., & Lewinsohn, P. (Eds.). (1986). *Geropsychological assessment and treatment: Selected topics.* New York: Springer.

Terracciano, A., & Costa, P. T. J. (2004). Smoking and the five-factor model of personality. *Addiction, 99,* 472–481.

Thompson, L. W., Gallagher, D., & Breckenridge, J. S. (1987). Comparative effectiveness of psychotherapies for depressed elders. *Journal of Consulting and Clinical Psychology, 55,* 385–390.

Tombaugh,T. N., & McIntyre, N. J. (1992). The Mini-Mental State Examination: A comprehensive review. *Journal of the American Geriatrics Society, 40,* 922–935.

Townsend, J., Adamo, M., & Haist, F. (2006). Changing channels: An fMRI study of aging and cross-modal attention shifts. *Neuroimage, 31,* 1682–1692.

Tuckman, B.W. (1965). Developmental sequence in small groups. *Psychological Bulletin, 63,* 384–399.

Tuckman, B. W., & Jensen, M. A. (1977). Stages of small group development revisited. *Group and Organization Studies, 2,* 419–427.

Tuleya, L. G. (2007). *Thesaurus of psychological index terms* (11th ed.). Washington, DC: American Psychological Association.

U.S. Bureau of the Census. (2007). *National population estimates – Characteristics.* Retrieved December 20, 2008, from //www.census.gov/popest/national/asrh/NC-EST2006-asrh. html.

U.S. Bureau of the Census. (2008). Facts for features: Grandparents Day 2008: September 7. Retrieved December 20, 2008, from www.census.gov/Press--release/www/releases/ archives/facts_for_features_special_editions/012095.html.

U.S. Department of Health and Human Services. (1999). *Mental health: A report of the Surgeon General.* Rockville, MD: U.S. Department of Health and Human Services, Substance Abuse and Mental Health Services Administration, Center for Mental Health Services, National Institutes of Health, National Institute of Mental Health.

U.S. Department of Health and Human Services. (2001). *National standards on culturally and linguistically appropriate services in health care from Office of Minority Health.* Rockville, MD: IQ Solutions. Retrieved December 20, 2008, from www.omhrc.gov/clas

U.S. Surgeon General. (1999). *Mental health: A report of the Surgeon General.* Retrieved February 8, 2008, from www.surgeongeneral.gov/library/mentalhealth/home.html.

Unützer, J., Katon, W., Callahan, C. M., Williams, J. W., Hunkeler, E., Harpoole, L., et al. (2002). Collaborative care management of late-life depression in the primary care setting: A randomized controlled trial. *JAMA, 288,* 2836–2845.

Vacha-Haase, T., & Duffy, M. (in press). Counseling psychologists working with an older adult population. In B. Altmaier and J. Hansen (Eds.), *Handbook of counseling psychology.* New York: Oxford University Press.

Van Manen, J. G., Bindels, P. J. E., Dekker, F. W., IJzermans, C., J., van der Zee, J. S., & Schade, E. (2002). Risk of depression in patients with chronic obstructive pulmonary disease and its determinants. *Thorax, 57,* 412–416.

van Schaik, A., van Marwijk, H., Ader, H., van Dyck, R., de Haan, M., Penninx, B., et al. (2008). Interpersonal psychotherapy for elderly patients in primary care. *American Journal of Geriatric Psychiatry, 14,* 777–786.

Van Solinge, H., & Henkens, K. (2008). Adjustment to and satisfaction with retirement: Two of a kind? *Psychology and Aging, 23,* 422–434.

Verdeli, H., Clougherty, K., Bolton, P., Speelman, L., Ndogoni, L., Bass, J., et al. (2003). Adapting group interpersonal psychotherapy for a developing country: Experience in rural Uganda. *World Psychiatry, 2,* 114–120.

Veterans Health Administration National Ethics Committee. (2007a). *Ethical aspects of the relationship between clinicians and surrogate decision makers.* Washington, DC: Veterans Health Administration.

Veterans Health Administration National Ethics Committee. (2007b). *Impaired driving in older adults: Ethical challenges for health care professionals.* Washington, DC: Veterans Health Administration.

Vig, E. K., Starks, H., Taylor, J. S., Hopley, E. K., & Fryer-Edwards, K. (2007). Surviving surrogate-decision making: What helps and hampers the experience of making medical decisions for others. *Society of General Internal Medicine, 22,* 1274–1279.

Volicer, L., Cantor, M. D., Derse, A. R., Edwards, D. M., Prudhomme, A. M., Gregory, D. C., et.al. (2002). Advance care planning by proxy for residents of long-term care facilities who lack decision-making capacity. *Journal of the American Geriatrics Society, 50*(4), 761–767.

Wagner, E. H., Bennett, S. M., Austin, B. T., Greene, S. M., Schaefer, J. K., & Vonkorff, M. (2005). Finding common ground: Patient-centeredness and evidence-based chronic illness care. *Journal of Alternative and Complementary Medicine, 11* Suppl 1, S7–15.

Walfish, S., & Barnett, J. E. (2009). *Financial success in mental health practice: Essential tools and strategies for practitioners.* Washington, DC: American Psychological Association.

Wan, H., Sengupta, M., Velkoff, V. A., & DeBarros, K. A. (2005). *U.S. Census Bureau, Current population reports, P23–209, 65+ in the United States: 2005.* Washington, DC: U.S. Government Printing Office.

Warr, P., Butcher, V., Robertson, I., & Callinan, M. (2004). Older people's well-being as a function of employment, retirement, environmental characteristics and role preference. *British Journal of Psychology, 95,* 297–324.

Watkins, C. E. (Ed.). (1997). *Handbook of psychotherapy supervision* (pp. 366–380). New York: John Wiley.

Weale, R. A. (1987). Senescent vision: Is it all the fault of the lens? *Eye, 1,* 217–221.

Weinberg, D. B., Gittell, J. H., Lusenhop, R. W., Kautz, C. M., & Wright J. (2007). Beyond our walls: impact of patient and provider coordination across the continuum on outcomes for surgical patients. *Health Services Research, 42*(1 Pt 1), 7–24.

Weissman, M. M., Markowitz, J. C., & Klerman, G. L. (2000). *Comprehensive guide to interpersonal psychotherapy.* New York: Basic Books.

Weissman, M. M., & Paykel, E. (1974). *The depressed woman.* Chicago: University of Chicago Press.

Wenger, N. S., Solomon, D. H., Roth, C. P., MacLean, C. H., Saliba, D., Kamberg, C. J., et al. (2003). The quality of medical care provided to vulnerable community-dwelling older patients. *Annals of Internal Medicine, 139*(9), 740–747.

Wetherell, J. L., LeRoux, H., & Gatz, M. (2003). *DSM-IV* criteria for generalized anxiety disorder in older adults: Distinguishing the worried from the well. *Psychology and Aging, 18,* 622–627.

Wetherell, J. L., Sorrell, J. T., Thorp, S. R., & Patterson, T. L. (2005). Psychological interventions for late-life anxiety: A review and early lessons from the CALM Study. *Journal of Geriatric Psychiatry and Neurology, 18,* 72–82.

Whitbourne, S. K. (1986). *The me I know: A study of adult identity.* New York: Springer-Verlag.

Whitbourne, S. K. (1996). *Division 20: Past and present perspective.* Washington, DC: Division 20.

Whitbourne, S. K. (2000). *Psychopathology in later adulthood.* New York: John Wiley.

Whitbourne, S. K. (2002). *The aging individual: Physical and psychological perspectives* (2nd ed.). New York: Springer.

Whitbourne, S. K., & Cavanaugh, J. C. (Eds.). (2003). *Integrating aging topics into psychology: A practical guide for teaching.* Washington, DC: American Psychological Association.

Whitbourne, S. K., & Collins, K. C. (1998). Identity and physical changes in later adulthood: Theoretical and clinical implications. *Psychotherapy, 35,* 519–530.

Whitbourne, S. K., Sneed, J. R., & Sayer, A. (2009). Psychosocial development from college through mdlife: A 34-year sequential study. *Developmental Psychology, 45*(5), 1328-1340.

Whitlatch, C. J., Feinberg, L. F., & Tucke, S. S. (2005). Measuring the values and preferences for everyday care of persons with cognitive impairment and their family caregivers. *The Gerontologist, 45*(3), 370–380.

Wilcox, S., Evenson, K. R., Aragaki, A., Wassertheil-Smoller, S., Mouton, C. P., & Loevinger, B. L. (2003). The effects of widowhood on physical and mental health, health behaviors, and health outcomes: The Women's Health Initiative. *Health Psychology, 22*, 513–522.

Wild, K., & Cotrell, V. (2003). Identifying driving impairment in Alzheimer disease: A comparison of self and observer reports versus driving evaluation. *Alzheimer Disease and Associated Disorders, 17*(1), 27–34.

Wilkins, C. H., Sheline, Y. I., Roe, C. M., Birge, S. J., & Morris, J. C. (2006). Vitamin D deficiency is associated with low mood and worse cognitive performance in older adults. *American Journal of Geriatric Psychiatry, 14*, 1032–1040.

Williams, J. B., Kobak, K. A., Bech, P., Engelhardt, N., Evans, K., Lipsitz, J., et al. (2008). The GRID-HAMD: Standardization of the Hamilton Depression Rating Scale. *International Clinical Psychopharmacology, 23*,120–129.

Williams, J. W. Jr., Katon, W., Lin, E. H., Noel, P. H., Worchel, J., Cornell, J., et al. (2004). IMPACT investigators. The effectiveness of depression care management on diabetes-related outcomes in older patients. *Annals of Internal Medicine, 140*(12), 1015–1024.

Willis, S. L., Tennstedt, S. L., Marsiske, M., Ball, K., Elias, J., Koepke, K. M., et al. (2006). Long-term effects of cognitive training on everyday functional outcomes in older adults. *JAMA, 296*, 2805–2814.

Wingfield, A., & Kahana, M. J. (2002). The dynamics of memory retrieval in older adulthood. *Canadian Journal of Experimental Psychology, 56*, 187–199.

Winzelberg, G. S., Hanson, L. C., & Tulsky, J. A. (2005). Beyond autonomy: Diversifying end-of-life decision-making approaches to serve patients and families. *Journal of the American Geriatrics Society, 53*(6), 1046–1050.

Wolff, J. L., & Roter, D. L. (2008). Hidden in plain sight: Medical visit companions as a resource for vulnerable older adults. *Archives of Internal Medicine, 168*, 1409–1415.

Wood, E. (2004). History of guardianship. In M. J. Quinn (Ed.), *Guardianships of adults: Achieving justice, autonomy, and safety* (pp. 17–48). New York: Springer.

Woodford, H. J., & George, J. (2007). Cognitive assessment in the elderly: A review of clinical methods. *QJM, 100*, 469–484.

Xakellis, G., Brangman, S. A., Hinton, W. L., Jones, V. Y., Masterman, D., Pan, C. X., et al. (2004). Curricular framework: Core competencies in multicultural geriatric care. *Journal of the American Geriatrics Society, 52*, 137–142.

Yalom, I. D. (2008). *Staring at the sun: Overcoming the terror of death.* San Francisco: Jossey-Bass.

Yang, F. M., & Levkoff, S. E. (2005, Fall). Ageism and minority populations: Strengths in the face of challenge. *Generations*, 42–48.

Yarry, S. J., Stevens, E. K., & McCallum, T. J. (2007, Fall). Cultural influences on spousal caregiving. *Generations*, 24–30.

Yeo, G., & Gallagher-Thompson, D. (Eds.). (2006). *Ethnicity and the dementias* (2nd ed.). New York: Routledge/Taylor & Francis.

Yesavage, J. A. (1988). Geriatric depression scale. *Psychopharmacology Bulletin, 24*, 709–710.

Yesavage, J. A., Brink, T. L., Rose, T. L., Lum, O., Huang, V., Adey, M., et al. (1983). Development and validation of a geriatric depression screening scale: A preliminary report. *Journal of Psychiatric Research, 17*(1), 37–49.

Yon, A., & Scogin (2007). Procedures for identifying evidence-based psychological treatments for older adults. *Psychology and Aging, 22,* 4–7.

Young, J., & Beck, A. (1980). *Cognitive Therapy Scale: Rating manual.* Unpublished manuscript, Center for Cognitive Therapy, Philadelphia, PA.

Zanetti, M. V., Cordeiro, Q., & Busatto, G. F. (2007). Late onset bipolar disorder associated with white matter hyperintensities: A pathophysiological hypothesis. *Progress in Neuropsychopharmacology and Biological Psychiatry, 31,* 551–556.

Zarit, S. (1980). *Aging and mental disorders.* New York: Free Press:

Zeiss, A. M., & Gallagher-Thompson, D. (2003). Providing interdisciplinary geriatric team care: What does it really take? *Clinical Psychology: Science and Practice, 10*(1), 115–119.

Zeiss, A., & Karlin, B. (2008). Integrating mental health and primary care services in the Department of Veterans Affairs health care system. *Journal of Clinical Psychology in Mental Health Settings, 15,* 73–78.

Zeiss, A. M., & Steffen. A. (1996). Interdisciplinary health care teams: The basic unit of geriatric care. In L. L. Carstensen, B. A. Edelstein, & L. Dornbrand (Eds.), *The handbook of clinical geropsychology* (pp. 423–450). Thousand Oaks, CA: Sage.

Zelinski, E. M., & Burnight, K. P. (1997). Sixteen-year longitudinal and time lag changes in memory and cognition in older adults. *Psychology and Aging, 12,* 503–513.

INDEX